A JOURNEY FROM FAT TO FLAT

How I Overcame Being Overweight -- And How You Can Do It, Too

By A'Cora Berry

A JOURNEY FROM FAT TO FLAT

TABLE OF CONTENTS

INTRODUCTION

A Journey from Fat to Flat tells my story of overcoming childhood sexual abuse and struggling with being overweight. Then, it shows how my experience can help others, whether they are dealing with similar issues or have other challenges to overcome.

Thus, while I begin with my own story, this book is designed to help others heal. As I describe, I initially kept my own abuse from seven to ten at the hands of a neighbor secret from my family, but when I finally stood up to him when I was 11, he no longer abused me. Even so, I still had to overcome the lingering effects, which included struggling with my weight. I went through a series of challenges and overcame them along the way.

This book also describes the strategies and techniques I used to finally overcome these problems. Then, it focuses on the techniques I learned for losing weight and building strength. These techniques can be used by anyone facing those particular issues and can be applied more broadly to other challenges one faces in life.

To this end, the book is divided into these sections:

- My journey and how I overcame my own struggles,
- The problem of overeating and how to overcome being overweight,
- Applying the techniques I used to any problems you are facing in your life,

The book concludes with some resources for further reading about the particular issues I dealt with -- experiencing sexual abuse and dealing with overeating and becoming overweight.

CHAPTER 1: MY JOURNEY

My journey to wanting to help others deal with the two major problems I faced in my life -- overcoming sexual abuse as a child and reducing my weight and becoming healthy again -- begins with my own struggles. I learned so much along the way that I want to share this with others.

My journey begins in Mexico, where I came from a big family. My first five years were very happy ones, growing up in a small town, where my mother and father were farmers, and my mother additionally did some odd jobs for extra income, such as washing laundry by hand for the neighbors to bring in extra income.

Though we were poor, my parents were very warm and loving, and I remember fun celebrations on major holidays and family events, including Independence Day festivals on September 16, las posadas navidenas celebrations in December, Quinceanera celebrations when a girl in our circle of relatives turned 15, and backyard barbecues. We had friendly and supportive neighbors, too, who were ready to help if our family needed anything.

For example, neighbors that used to have a small grocery store let my mother pay credit for groceries, because we were very poor. Another neighbor with a little clothes store let my mother pay on credit for our clothes, when we bought new clothes once a year for the Fiesta del Pueblo celebration. We only bought new clothes at this time and bought second-hand clothes at other times, because we couldn't afford new ones. Another neighbor, who was my godmother, sometimes took me with her to their family home in the city, and sometimes she took me to a concert and a restaurant.

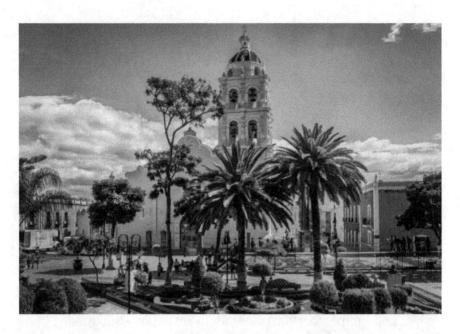

I was also a very playful and joyful girl. I used to play with some other children in the neighborhood until late at night. I went for bike rides with my friends, and I loved to chase turtles at the small stream by my house. Sometimes when my mother worked on farming our land, I went to the stream to look for shrimp.

When Everything Changed

When I was five, everything changed. My father had an argument with a friend who shot him in the back, and he died instantly. I remember that I was wearing a yellow dress that my grandmother made for me, which was like sunlight. But now darkness descended on me and the family.

That night, my mother, my two brothers, who were 11 and 17, and my three sisters, who were 9, 13 and 15, went to a memorial for my father at my grandmother's house, and the living room was filled with people, who hugged each other, sobbed, and shared stories of what a good man my father had been. My two other older sisters weren't able to attend, since they were living in the United States.

8

That terrible night was the first time I saw my mother cry, and I sobbed with her. I was in shock, feeling the great loss of my father and wondering how such a devastating thing could happen so unexpectedly. It was like the hand of God suddenly reached down and took someone away. My brothers were emotionally destroyed, too. Meanwhile, my father's friend had been taken to jail by the local police, and people talked about how sad it is when a one-time friend becomes an enemy or harms a good friend.

Over the next few days, my mother tried to be strong. She dried her tears and tried to appear very strong to us children, as she became a mother and father figure to all of us. Yet I imagine that inside she was dying from her deep suffering, and the strength she showed outwardly was to let us know that everything would be okay.

Now, instead of my father, she became the family provider, and she did everything she could to put food on the table. She worked as a farmer, though sometimes there wasn't much to do, so she did odd jobs, such as doing the laundry for neighbors. I remember seeing her wash by hand huge loads of laundry for the neighbors to make ends meet. Sometimes she also worked at night for a fruit processing company. Managing after my father died was especially hard for her, because she only finished elementary school, so many jobs were closed to her. But she did the best she could.

Meanwhile, over the years, she didn't speak any more about my father's death, and so neither did I. Yet his death hung over us like an unseen ghost, since we never spoke about our grievances and feelings.

A Loss of Innocence

When I was 7, another incident that shocked my world happened when I was sexually molested by a neighbor. What he did happened so unexpectedly. I was at his house while I was visiting his daughter. I think he lured me into a bedroom and shut the door, though my memory of exactly how he got me alone is very foggy.

9

Before I knew it, he was touching me under my clothes, and afterwards he told me to never tell my mother, since she wouldn't believe me and bad things would happen.

When it was over and I rejoined my friend, I felt shocked and ashamed. I didn't say anything, because I was just a little girl, and I was afraid that my mother wouldn't believe me or that my neighbor would do something to hurt my mother or the rest of the family in some way. I was especially afraid he might harm my mother, since I had recently lost my father, and I didn't want anything bad to happen to her. So I said nothing, and from time to time, my neighbor would get me alone in his house and touch me again.

These encounters with my neighbor went on for about four years, and I quietly endured them, afraid to say anything. Meanwhile, this experience affected me in the way I was with other kids, especially with boys in my school. I felt distant and different from others, so it was hard to communicate with them, and I certainly didn't want to say anything about my neighbor. I thought they might say I teased or flirted with him or did something to attract him. So I felt very much the victim.

But finally, when I was 11, I felt enough was enough. Maybe somehow that time when he tried to touch me, it was the last straw. I just didn't want to give in and be the victim anymore. I don't know what happened to give me this strength to resist, but whatever the reason, I did so one day when I was in my house, and he came up from behind my back. When he tried to touch my body, I was indignant, pulled away, and told him: "Do not touch me again, you son of a bitch." At once he pulled away, and he never touched me again.

After that happened, I felt liberated, like I had finally broken free of the man who abused me, like I was a bird escaping its cage. Yet at the same time, because of what happened, I started to distrust people in general.

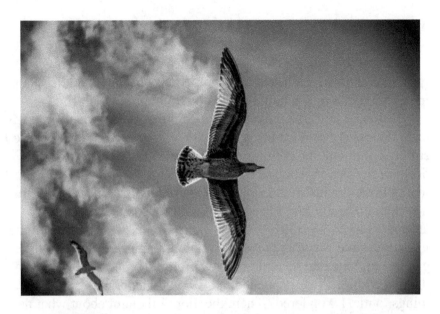

    Contributing to my distrust, I never talked about what happened with my family. Perhaps my reaction would have been different, given what I have since learned, if I had told them. But back then, I didn't understand what I know now is that your body is like a temple, and no one has a right to touch or enter it, unless you give them the permission to do so, such as you might do with a significant other or husband. Thus, maybe if I had had that conversation with my mother when I was child, I would have had the knowledge and strength to stop the abuse in the very beginning. But I didn't, and that is one reason I think it is so important to share this information about maintaining one's boundaries with one's children early on.

    Now I have two young daughters, and as soon as they were old enough to understand at seven or eight, I told them the importance of taking care of their bodies and rejecting any inappropriate advances. I wished I could have had that conversation with my mother, but that is long in the past, so there is nothing I can do now except to be better than my mother in preparing my daughters, so they can do better than me.

Turnaround

The third major change in my life centered around my weight, and how I dealt with the problem has become another plank in my approach to teaching people how to improve their life.

I experienced a major weight gain that began when I was 13 to 14. Looking back, I think it had a lot to do with the sexual abuse I suffered and with the continuing emptiness I felt due to the early death of my father. Though I had once been a playful and happy girl, that outlook gradually faded away. I started by isolating myself from my closest friends, and I became even more isolated, when I was around 13 and a so-called "family friend" in his 30s approached me in a suggestive way that is inappropriate for approaching a young girl. He told me that he realized how pretty I looked and had sexual dreams with me. I was shocked. How could he possibly say those things to me, I wondered? Then, the more I thought about what he said, the more devastated I felt. I wondered if that was the way other men looked at me. After that, I wanted to conceal myself and not attract attention. I also felt that not having a male figure in my life made me more vulnerable to predators, and I think I was more receptive to responding this way because of the lingering sadness from my father's death. At the same time, I knew I would stand up for myself should any other men speak to me inappropriately in the future.

In any case, after that approach from a family friend got me reflecting about the earlier abuse I experienced, I started to feel less confident and more self-conscious, so I started to overeat because it made me feel better. I had larger portions during my meals and ate more snacks during the day, and much of this extra food consisted of pastries and candies, because they tasted so good. Then, for a little time after each meal or snack, I felt good. It was like I got a boost from a sugar high.

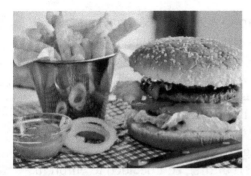 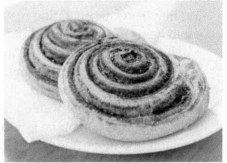

But after the high ended, my spirits would sink, and I would look for another infusion of extra food to bring back that joy. Then, after a few weeks of overeating, my weight began to climb markedly, and I felt sad, because I was putting all that extra weight on my body. My initial reaction was to simply eat more food, especially sweet food, to feel better again. It was like I was stuck in a vicious cycle, and I couldn't get out as my weight jumped from 120 to 140 to 160 and eventually to 220 pounds. I couldn't stop, because overeating led me to feel a brief surge of happiness. Then, that was followed by sadness which led me to overeat again.

The cycle continued through my teenage years and into my 20s. By the time I was in my early 30s and weighted so much, I thought I would be overweight for the rest of my life.

So how could I stop the spiral, where my weight went up and my spirits plunged down? I felt truly stuck.

Then, everything changed one day when I was watching an Oprah Winfrey show, and I heard her talking about childhood sexual abuse. That moment was very liberating for me, because until that moment I kept the molestation a secret. The only person who I told about it was my husband, who I married when I was in my 20s.

But now, seeing all of these women who were molested when they were young and were now willing to talk about it was very liberating. I realized what had happened to me wasn't my fault, because I had been a young child, so I was vulnerable when an older neighbor I considered a family friend had attacked me. As a result of this program, I felt like a huge weight was lifted from my shoulders, and I wasn't as mad at myself or distrustful of others as I had been. I

13

felt like the wall separating me from others melted away, and now I could be open and honest about what happened to me, so I could speak freely about the past. Thus, I felt truly liberated, and I wanted to share my new understandings with others.

Then, this feeling of release led me to want to stop overeating, too. Plus I wanted to have a healthy weight as an example to my daughters. I didn't want them to follow my example by eating too much and becoming overweight like me.

I didn't know where to start at first, so I decided to enroll in the local YMCA. I told my husband what I wanted to do, and he was very encouraging. "Go do it. You can do it," he told me.

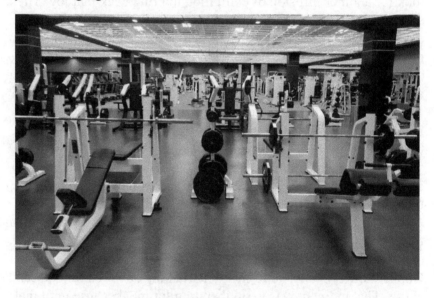

The YMCA had a class on losing weight, which I attended along with a dozen other women. I felt inspired by being with the other people in the class to commit myself to a program to lose weight. Then, based on the advice of the instructor, I began spending 30 minutes a day walking and another 30 minutes lifting small 5 pound weights. Gradually, I worked up to heavier 10 and 15 pound weights.

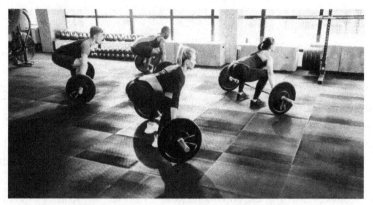

At first, I felt very uncomfortable lifting these weights. Because I was so heavy at 224 pounds when I began this new regimen, I got very tired after even 15 minutes of exertion, such as when I went to the store to get groceries. Now, just trying to walk or lift weights for 30 minutes each day got me very tired. After about 10 minutes of each activity, I wanted to quit. Even before I started exercising, my mind would make excuses to get me to stop, such as telling me: "You're too tired...You're too busy...It's raining outside...It's too cold."

But my attitude changed in one of my group classes, after I saw some women really pushing themselves. I even met women who had recently had surgeries and were already pushing themselves to be healthier. So I urged myself to go on. "Just do it," I told myself. "You'll be healthier. You'll feel better if you keep going." So I did.

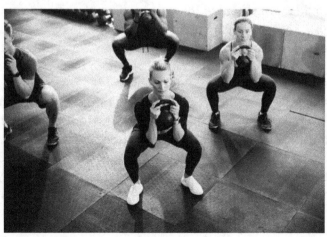

Then, gradually, I found I could walk or lift weights for a longer and longer time, which is what happens when you try to break any new habit and increase your endurance. It is a very hard struggle at first to keep trying to break the habit, but as the days, weeks, and months go by, it becomes easier and easier to make the break. You just need your commitment in the beginning to push through and keep going. So that's what I did. I kept pushing away that screaming in my head that said: "Stop doing this. Quit. Take it easy. Relax," and I pressed on. I knew I needed to do this exercising to live a healthier active life.

For further inspiration, I began reading books about losing weight and becoming healthy, too. In one of them, reinforcing my commitment to exercise more, I found a quote that helped to motivate me: "The person that wants to do something finds a way; the other finds an excuse." I even wrote the quote on a piece of paper and put it on my car's dashboard, so I could look at it every day when I got in the car as a reminder to keep going. The quote also helped me think about the importance of the small steps one takes that eventually lead to a goal. As the quote reminded me, you should never underestimate anything that you're doing to accomplish your goal. It doesn't matter how small your efforts are, the little efforts make the big goals possible.

Thus, such ideas helped to keep me inspired and motivated, as I worked to lose weight and eat a more healthy diet. As I did, I found I could do many more things. For example, after a very busy day at work, I was able to take on more chores at home. I found I needed less sleep, too, so I was able to be very active after a good night's sleep -- only six hours for me, although others may find that seven or eight hours works best for them.

Along the way, I also learned some of the most important principles about doing this weight loss successfully, such as eating a healthy breakfast, engaging in effective strength training, and understanding how the body burns sugar, fats, and proteins. I began to learn these principles when I discovered that, despite all my exercising and feeling less tired, I wasn't losing weight at first. But that's because my muscles were getting stronger, and they weighed more than the fat in my originally fat flabby arms, so I weighed more while my body slimmed down.

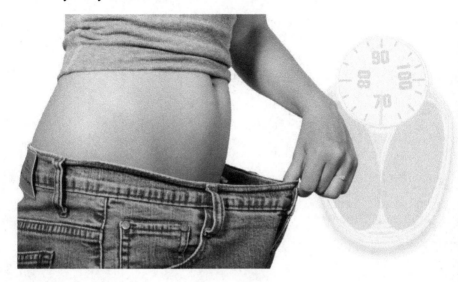

Thus, I realized it's necessary to apply certain principles to both lose weight and get stronger, and that's what I'll talk about in the next chapters -- what I learned you should do to both curb your overeating and lose weight in an effective way. I have included some photos to illustrate these various health tips and techniques.

CHAPTER 2: WHAT I LEARNED ABOUT LOSING WEIGHT AND LIVING A HEALTHY LIFE

Here I want to briefly describe my experience in learning to exercise and lift weights for strength in order to burn off calories effectively. Then, I will discuss each of these topics in more details.

This experience began in my early 30s, when I was extremely overweight and felt little energy both on my job as a customer service rep and at home with my family. At first, I was in denial about how heavy I was. On one occasion I even told my mother that the weight on the scales was all wrong, since it wasn't possible for me to be that heavy. But she quickly put down my response with her brutally honest response. "The weights are not wrong. You're definitely overweight."

Thus, I had to face the fact that I had become very overweight. Then, I felt inspired to change after hearing Oprah's program on how people can change if they commit themselves and set personal goals. After that I began reading different books and articles on what to do about reducing my weight and gaining more energy. I found many articles by searching on Google.

Discovering the Power of Exercise

In the beginning, when I was very overweight at about 220 pounds, my arms were huge, so I was very concerned about concealing them. Accordingly, whenever I got dressed, I put something on to cover them, like a sweater. Even it was hot outside, I wore one. I was very self-conscious and my self-esteem was way down. But as I started exercising and losing weight, my arms began getting smaller and smaller, and I felt good about the changes.

It's hard to separate the different things I did, since I started doing everything once I joined the YMCA and went to their gym where I took classes and lifted weights. I also began eating a more nutritious breakfast in the morning and going for longer and longer walks. Thus, while I will talk about each of these elements separately in the following chapters, you may want to do them at the same time, as I did, which is ideal, since one activity will reinforce another. But if you prefer, you can do these things separately, such as if you start going on walks without lifting weights or just change your eating habits, including eating a healthy breakfast.

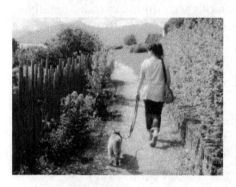 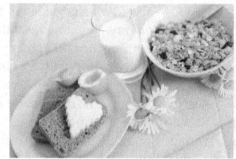

You may find you experience some resistance to making these changes, as I did. It was hard to change when I first started. For example, while I hoped to walk 30 minutes a day, when I started, I didn't have that much energy when I was walking. Even if I walked for only 15 minutes, I would feel very tired, although now I can easily run for five miles and run for 90 minutes. Thus, I gradually increased the distance and time I ran little by little. Every week or two, I would add a few more minutes and run a little further. As I did more miles, I ran faster, too.

You might plan to do the same by gradually increasing what you do to exercise. Expect to begin slowly, so you down tire yourself out. Then, do a little more to stretch your ability each day, whether it's walking, which is good for your cardio, or weight lifting, which builds your muscles and strength. You can even enjoy walking with a friend, and if you have a child, you can take him or her along.

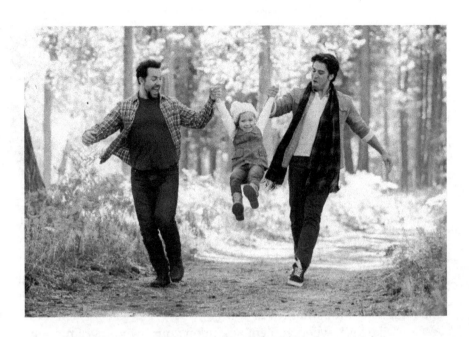

I had the same experience in going to the gym. I felt determined to get in shape, so I kept telling myself: "You have to go. You have to go." But I was pushing myself in the beginning, because I often didn't want to go, especially when I was very tired from work, or I had to get up early on Saturday morning to go to the gym before other activities for the day. Thus, I often told myself excuses to avoid going, such as saying to myself "I don't want to go; it's raining" or "I don't feel like it." But then I would resist my resistance and tell myself: "No, I have to go. I've got to go."

Once I was at the gym and started to work out, I felt better. That's because as soon as I started lifting the weights, I felt my energy and strength increase. I felt more focused and directed. So my spirits lifted, and I ended up having a great workout. Afterwards, I felt very proud of myself for pushing myself to be there and work out, even though I didn't want to be there initially. Likewise, once you start exercising regularly, you will feel your mind kick in, so you focus on whatever you are doing. You will also feel a charge of energy that will give you a mental boost.

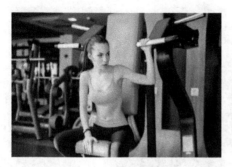 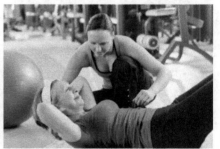

Aside from my determination to lose weight and feel better, I got encouragement from my husband and family, which contributed to my continued commitment. I remember going to family gatherings where the members of my family would say: "This is cool. She's doing something for herself." So I felt a sense of pride at these gatherings. They were a place to show off my progress and get encouragement for what I was doing.

Likewise, when you embark upon your own program, look to others in your circle of family members and friends to gain their praise and support. If you feel a need for even more support, you can find support groups through your gym, church, or other community networks.

Fortunately, I didn't have any relapses, though I know that sometimes happens to people going through these programs. They get tired and put off exercising, so one day becomes two, then three, and longer, and it can feel hard to start again. But if you feel like pausing for a time, one day off is fine for you to relax. But after that, if you feel resistance coming up, you have to push yourself to keep going. Then, once you start exercising and working out again, that feeling of energy will come back to inspire you to stay on track.

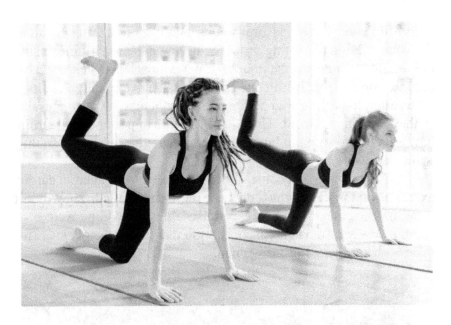

I found that my energy and moods kept getting better and better, so now I'm always very smiley and happy and feel more energy. Additionally, over the months when I began exercising and eating better, I noticed I could do much more both at work and with my kids and other family members, and I still had energy to do more. So I thought to myself: "Oh, wow! This is great," because before then, I was often tired and wasn't doing as much. In turn, noticing the difference helped inspire me to keep going and do even more.

By the same token, pay attention to how you feel and what you do, as you engage in your own exercise and eat healthy program. This recognition of your accomplishments will help you feel even more confident and committed to what you are doing.

I also found it helpful to talk to other women who were lifting weights, too, at the gym. I found they became a kind of support community, since we were all going through the same process together in seeking to lose weight, build strength, or both. At the same time, it was a learning experience to realize that not all of the women were doing the exercises correctly. For example, one woman complained that her arms were still flaccid after she had been lifting weights for several weeks. But it soon became apparent she wasn't doing the lifting properly, because she wasn't increasing the weights to increase the pressure on her muscles. Instead, she had become comfortable lifting one of the smaller five pound weights. As a result, the lifting was no longer strengthening her arm muscles, so they remained flaccid. Thus, I realized the importance of learning how to do these strength building exercises in the right way, so they will be effective.

I also found that some of the women who engaged in cardio exercises on the treadmills didn't use the weights at all. They didn't want to, since they thought the exercises they were doing were enough. Many also had a misconception that lifting weights was for male body builders, not for women.

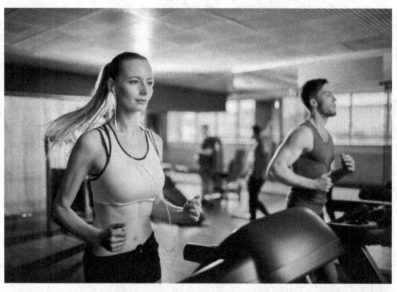

To counter their resistance, I urged them to lift the weights, explaining that building up the muscles in the body is not just for men. Then, I told them: "Working with the weights is going to make you feel good. Just try it." I also told them that it's important to do this lifting for your body, because as you lose weight, you want to tighten your skin. Otherwise, it will remain flaccid or hang even more, because as you lose weight, if you don't build up your muscles, your skin will sag." I also explained how lifting weights worked for me, because I may have weighed more than they did when I started, but my arms became tight because I was lifting weights since the beginning. I found many of the women I spoke to very receptive to my suggestions, and they began lifting weights, too.

Another advantage I found in lifting weights is it made me feel very relaxed. Sometimes when I run, I don't get that feeling. But when I lift weights, it relaxes me. Perhaps it does so, because I can stay focused on the process of lifting and even close my eyes when doing it. By contrast, when I run I have to pay attention to the environment around me in order to stay on the trail or street when I am outside, and I have to be careful not to run into someone. In any case, experiencing that feeling of relaxation is another benefit of lifting weights which I have explained to other women.

Then, too, I found that these changes in your weight and strength take time, and that can be discouraging at first. Even though I soon began to feel more energy and more relaxed during the workout sessions, I didn't notice any changes for a couple of months. So I began asking some of the other women at the gym who I thought were in good shape how they did it. I went over to them while they were lifting weights or had just finished their regimen, and I told them: "I'm not seeing anything. I've been trying to build my strength, lose weight, and build up my muscles, but nothing seems to be happening. I don't know why." Then, the women I spoke to reassured me, telling me: "You know what? It takes time. So don't stop."

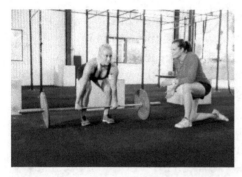 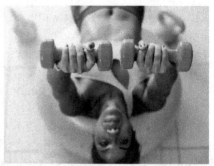

     Those words were encouraging to me, and now that I have achieved my goal of losing weight, building muscle, feeling more energy, and feeling better about myself, I have used what these women told me as another example of why those starting a workout regimen need to continue. They can't expect to see results right away. They have to realize that they are working for long-term changes that will take some time to achieve. And then they have to keep going to maintain their desired results.

     One more way to build a better body is using Pilates in addition to lifting weights to build strength. I started using this method about a year ago to shape my ab muscles and improve my posture. This type of exercise made me feel very good, so I kept doing it, and I go twice a week to a Pilates class, and I just love it. I also recommend Pilates because apart from ab building, it's another way to experience a sense of community with others in your class. Later, if you do the exercises on your own, you will find others at the gym who are doing this by themselves, so you can work out together. You can buy Pilates DVDs on Amazon or at Best Buy, or you can watch videos on YouTube.

Recognizing the Importance of Eating Right

Along with exercising, I changed my eating habits, so I ate healthier, nutritious foods, which are very important for any program of losing weight. You have to not only reduce the number of calories you take in, but increase the nutrition value of the foods you eat. In my case, I have become a vegetarian in the last few months, so I eat of lot of vegetables, including beans, avocados, and rice, and I try not to eat a lot of saturated foods, though otherwise I eat what I like. But you don't have to be a vegetarian to eat a better diet. The point is to reduce the sugars and carbs you eat, because those contribute to your putting on pounds.

I also found it important to stick to the diet each week, although I allowed a little leeway for special occasions, which you can do, too. For example, eating oatmeal has been a staple of my breakfast since I started a better eating regimen, which includes beginning the day with a healthy breakfast. I include oatmeal five or six days a week. But sometimes if my daughter wants to make something special for breakfast, I skip the oatmeal, so I can join her and my family. I do this because my daughter loves to cook, and sometimes she will make French toast on the weekend and at times for a special occasion, such as Mother's Day. Then, I will not have my oatmeal but will have her French toast, just for that day.

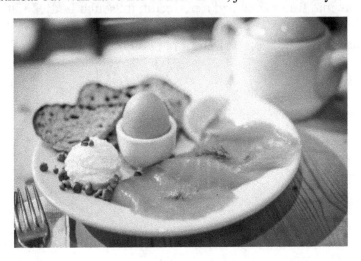

Thus, it's important if you are changing your eating habits to eat a healthier diet to allow for some flexibility. Mostly, you want to stick to the new diet, but from time to time, it's okay to relax and treat yourself to eating something else, such as for a family celebration. But don't overdo it and allow this break to open the door to abandoning your healthier diet. Just be selective and keep any break of your healthier diet to once a week.

Understanding How Your Body Burns Fuel

When I first started exercising, lifting weights, and eating right, I didn't understand anything about how the body burns sugar, fats, and proteins, so I left some foods that weren't very good for me in my diet. Then, I learned that knowing how the body burns calories is important for figuring on the best diet for you. Otherwise, you may not lose the weight or build the muscle you expect, if you are not following the right diet and weightlifting regimen.

My lesson in how the body burns fuel resulted from the very simple matter of adding cream to my coffee. When I started on my new weight loss and strength building regimen, I used to love creamer in my coffee. Though I had been regularly exercising for a month, I noticed that I wasn't losing weight, so I spoke to my friend, who was into fitness and had a powerful, muscular body. I told him, "It's been a month, and I noticed that I'm not losing weight." In response, he asked me: "Tell me what you do."

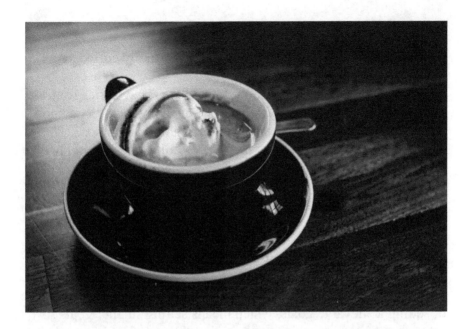

I described what I ate and the exercises I was practicing. He looked thoughtful and then asked me: "What about what you drink? And what do you put in it?" I told him "I have my coffee and I add creamer. I love my creamer."

That's when my friend explained the principles of burning fuel in your body. As he told me, "You know, by putting in creamer, you aren't giving your body the chance to burn what you already have. You're burning what you're consuming for fuel, but you're not burning what your body already has."

Why is that, I wondered, and he explained. "Your body burns off your sugars first, so you are loading up your body with extra sugars which it burns first. Or let me explain it this way: if you're putting in 400 calories of sugar with the creamer, and you are doing these various activities to lose weight, you are burning those 400 calories. But you will still have the same extra pounds in your body. You are just burning what you are consuming. You are not giving the body the opportunity to burn what it already has."

His explanation clicked for me. So little by little, I started cutting the creamer. I was not very happy about doing this, because I love the cream in my coffee. But over time, I cut the creamer down to nothing, and now I don't have any creamer in my coffee, and I'm fine with it.

Soon after his explanation, I heard the same stories from many other women in the gym. They would complain: "You know what? I'm exercising but I cannot lose weight. I cannot lose size." Then, they would tell me what they were eating, and I would realize they were making the same mistake that I made. So I would explain the basic principle. The body first burns glucose or sugar first, before it burns fats.

Setting Achievable Goals

After a few months of working out, I realized the importance of setting achievable goals, which means setting smaller goals so you can realistically achieve them rather than much larger goals that are harder to attain. When you do that, you might be discouraged from continuing towards a goal, because you haven't met your timeline for achieving it.

I realized that principle of setting smaller stepping stone goals, because when I first started on my journey, I wanted to lose 80 to 90 pounds. So I started to focus on losing the first 20 pounds. But I felt overwhelmed, because that goal didn't happen fast enough. I felt discouraged, too, and wondered if what I was doing was worth the effort.

Then, I spoke to a few people at the gym who were working on losing weight, and they told me how they set short-term goals for themselves. As a result, I told myself: "You know what? I'm going to lose five pounds." Then, I lost those five pounds and felt good, rather than feeling discouraged, because I hadn't come anywhere near to achieving my 20 pound goal.

Thus, setting these smaller goals was more encouraging to me. I know everyone is different, and some people may feel motivated by having a big goal -- sometimes referred to as an "audacious" goal, and later having a big celebration on achieving that milestone. But to me, focusing on a little bit at a time worked better than focusing on the very big goal.

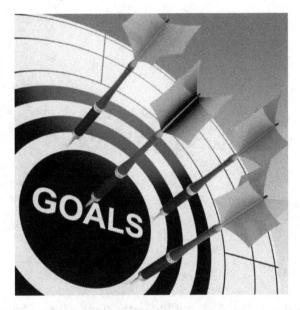

Likewise, though I wanted to lose 10 sizes, I told myself "No, no. Let me lose little by little." So I sought to drop one size at a time, and each time I did, I felt good. Then, that little by little approach led to my achieving a bigger and bigger accomplishment.

This kind of approach is much like that used to set up and work to achieve any goal. It helps to keep you motivated when you break the larger goal into sub goals or steps and mark your achievement along the way. This is the kind of approach advocated by business leaders and motivational experts. And this approach works well when you are seeking to lose weight, reduce your dress size, build up your muscles, or accomplish anything else. The key is to set measurable smaller goals and mark your achievement as you accomplish each one which brings you closer and closer to the last goal in the series. At the same time, give yourself some recognition and praise along the way; perhaps celebrate each achievement with a spouse, family members, or friends. The idea is to acknowledge yourself and your achievement and have others support what you have accomplished -- and that recognition will help you stay motivated and keep going to achieve your ultimate goal.

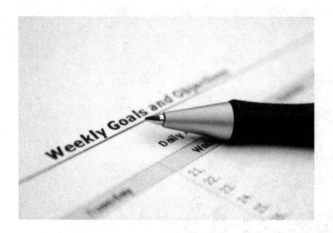 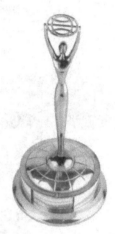

What's Next?

Now that I have laid out the basic steps which I have learned through my workout program, I want to go through each of these steps in more detail. I want to discuss more specifically the guidelines for starting your day with a good breakfast, building your body and strength through lifting weights, and understanding how your body burns sugars, fats, and proteins. Then, you can apply that knowledge in determining your diet.

I know there are many types of diet and workout programs, and if you are on one or more of these, fine. If it's working for you, keep doing it. What I want to do here is give you the basic principles and underlying research about why these methods work. Then, you can apply them to whatever programs you are currently on, if any.

The next chapters in this section cover these three topics:
- Eating right by starting with a healthy breakfast;
- Lifting weights effectively to build your body and your strength the right way;
- Knowing how to burn sugar, fats, and proteins, so you can adjust your diet accordingly.

CHAPTER 3: THE BENEFITS OF EATING A GOOD BREAKFAST

I previously described eating a good breakfast as one of the three key pillars of my program to lose weight and build strength. Now I want to describe in more detail why it is important to eat a good breakfast and how to do this.

Why Eat a Good Breakfast?

There are multiple reasons for starting the day with a breakfast, rather than waiting until lunchtime or satiating your hunger with some snacks to give you a burst of energy.

1) <u>Eating a nutritional breakfast can help you keep your weight down, since you are less likely to get hungry and eat more later</u>. Most scientists agree that if you haven't had breakfast, you are more likely to feel hungry and make up for it by eating more later during the day. Or without having breakfast, you might be more likely to pick up an unhealthy snack food to fill you up, such as grabbing a calorie filled snack bar or donut. By contrast, breakfast fills you up before you become very hungry, so you are less likely to grab whatever foods are available when you suddenly become hungry, such eating as a high energy, high fat protein bar, which has added sugar and salt.

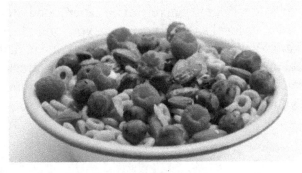

Another advantage of having a good breakfast is that you are more likely to get the vitamins, minerals, and other nutrients you need to build your body, so you need to eat less to get them, and that contributes to weight loss, too. For example, researchers have found this strong link between not eating breakfast and obesity. According to a BBC article: "Is Breakfast Really the Most Important Meal of the Day?" scientists in a U.S. study analyzed the health data of 50,000 people over seven years, and they found that those who made breakfast the largest meal of the day were more likely to have a lower BMI (body mass index) than those who ate a large lunch of dinner. Why? The researchers discovered that eating a healthy breakfast helps you feel satiated, so you reduce your daily calorie intake. Then, too, you are likely to have a higher quality diet, since breakfast foods are often higher in fiber and nutrients. Still another advantage of eating a good breakfast is that you improve your insulin sensitivity at your subsequent meals, so you are less likely to become diabetic or pre-diabetic.[1]

2) <u>You will keep your blood sugar level steadier during the day by preventing large fluctuations in your blood glucose level</u>. This steadiness helps you control your appetite. This benefit isn't only for those who have diabetes or a pre-diabetes condition. That's because maintaining this steady level can also help prevent diabetes, since it will help you avoid insulin resistance, which can be a precursor to diabetes. Maintaining this steady level is also an advantage, since if your blood sugar level goes down because you haven't had breakfast, or if it goes up and down when you supercharge it with a snack to increase your energy, this effect on your blood sugar level can negatively affect your mood. For example, when your level suddenly goes up, you might feel more nervous, anxious, irritable, or angry. Or if it goes down, that can make you feel tired, too. You might even feel more serious symptoms, such as having an irregular heartbeat or seizures, when the sugar in your blood is too low.

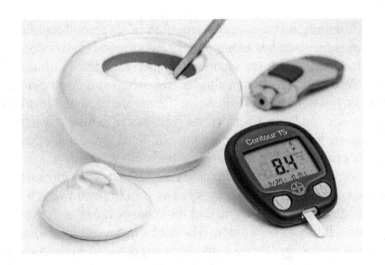

3) <u>You will keep down your blood glucose level</u>, which is important to avoid weight gain and the risk of getting diabetes. As reported in the BBC.com article, another study that used a randomized control group with 18 people with diabetes and 18 people without found that skipping breakfast disrupted the circadian rhythm of both groups. Skipping breakfast also resulted in larger spikes in the subjects' blood glucose levels after eating. Thus, the scientists concluded that having a good breakfast was essential to keep the body clock running on time.

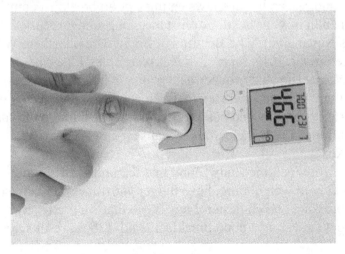

You might compare this situation of skipping breakfast to what happens when a watch's battery runs slow. It slows down, so the watch gradually loses seconds and then minutes, until it finally stops. Your body reacts in a similar way when you don't get the nutrients you need. You slow down, feel more tired, are less able to stay focused, and don't perform as well, because, like a watch mechanism, your body is running down, until you get another charge of nutrition that repairs your body clock again.

As expert Courtney Peterson explains it, your circadian clock has two parts -- one part is a master clock in the brain which is like the conductor of an orchestra, and the other part exists in every organ which has its own clock. These clocks are set by two key factors: your eating schedule and your exposure to light. As a result, if you eat at a time when you aren't being exposed to bright light, the clocks controlling your metabolism are in different time zones, which confuse the body, because it gets different signals indicating whether to rev up with bright light or power down with the low light condition. That's why it's better to eat that first meal for breakfast early when it's daylight, so you get a consistent signal for your body to rev up. Otherwise, as Peterson states, "eating late impairs blood sugar and blood pressure levels,"[2] since the lighting level is lower.

4) <u>You will have a healthier heart</u>. In this case,, scientists have found research that shows eating a good breakfast contributes to the health of your heart. For instance, one study, reported by Dennis Newman in "The Benefits of Eating Breakfast" on WebMD, appeared in the 2017 *Journal of the American College of Cardiology*. The study found that "people who skip breakfast are more likely to have atherosclerosis," a condition that occurs when your arteries narrow and harden because of the buildup of plaque. This buildup is very dangerous. because it can lead to a heart attack or stroke.

Moreover, the study found that the breakfast skippers were more likely to weigh more, have bigger waistlines, and have higher blood pressure and cholesterol levels. So that's a pretty strong argument for eating a good breakfast. And if those results are not convincing enough, another study found that individuals who skipped breakfast were more likely to have heart disease, smoke, drink more alcohol, and exercise less. In other words, skipping breakfast can be linked to a lot of unhealthy habits that contribute to heart problems, as well as to weight gain.

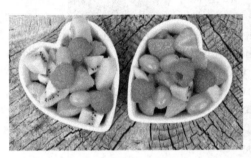 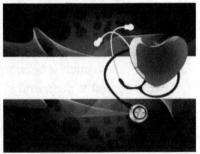

5) <u>You will have more brainpower, so you will be more effective in your work or at school</u>. Another reason that scientists agree on is that having a better breakfast is better, because it kick-starts your metabolism, so you have more energy and enthusiasm for what you are doing at work or in school. As a result, you will be better able to pay attention, concentrate, and remember things, which will help you do whatever you are doing more effectively. The reason you can perform so much better is because if you don't have breakfast, you have a lower energy level This leads your brain to slow down everything in your body, so it goes into what's called a "conservation mode." As a result, with this lower energy level, you may feel sluggish and have to struggle to maintain your concentration, because your brain hasn't received the necessary energy in the form of glucose to operate effectively.

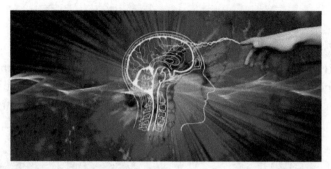

This slow-down is a little like what happens when a warm-blooded animal hibernates for the winter. Everything slows down so the animal uses much less energy. Your body doesn't close down to that extreme, but it goes into slow gear, like an auto going past a "slow down" sign. You don't have to stop, but you have to go more slowly, until you are ready to step on the gas -- like putting more energy into your body -- to go forward again.

6) <u>You will have more energy for whatever you are doing</u>. You will not only be more effective in whatever you are doing because you have more energy, but this extra energy will help you feel better. You will feel more alert and energetic. You will feel happier and joyful. Things won't bother you as much. You especially need this extra energy in the morning, because you haven't eaten for seven or more hours, and your body uses up energy while you sleep. As reported in a BBC.com article citing the writing of dietician Sarah Elder, "the body uses a lot of energy stores for growth and repair through the night. Eating a balanced breakfast helps to up your energy, as well as (provide more) protein and calcium used throughout the night."

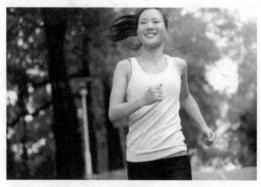

Another way to think of this increase in energy due to an early breakfast is to recognize that breakfast is a key to jumpstarting your metabolism. According to Fredrik Karp, a professor of metabolic medicine at the Oxford Center for Diabetes, Endocrinology, and Metabolism, as reported in the BBC.com article, you need an initial trigger involving carbs responding to insulin for your other tissues in your body to respond well to food intake. Having a good breakfast is critical to make this happen.

7) <u>You will be less likely to fall ill</u>. As researchers have found, those who regularly eat a good breakfast commonly have a lower risk of not only obesity and type 2 diabetes, but they are less likely to suffer from cardiovascular disease.

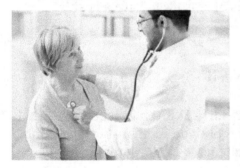 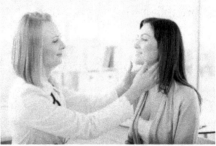

8) <u>You will tend to make better food choices</u>. As researchers have found, people who eat a good breakfast tend to eat a healthier diet the rest of the day, have better eating habits, and are less likely to become hungry and eat snacks during the day that those who don't have breakfast. By contrast, breakfast skippers often eat snacks during the mid-morning or afternoon, and often they make poor snacks choices, because they choose snacks that are high in fats and salt, such as the popular protein snack bars. While these bars are promoted as healthy nutritious foods, they are filled with nuts, chocolate, or other tasty treats, so they are more like candy bars than food supplements, and they commonly are low in fiber, vitamins, and minerals.

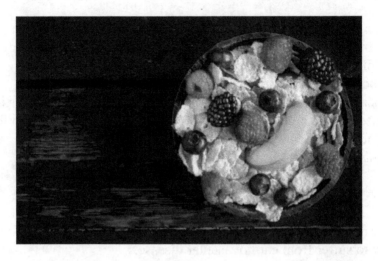

In sum, there are all kinds of reasons to have a healthy breakfast to start your day.

Studies that Support the Need for a Good Breakfast

Besides the reasons I have already given to support the need for a good breakfast, many studies provide additional evidence for eating right, not just to lose weight but to keep your body in tip-top shape.

For example, one study shows that if you skip breakfast, you have a 27% increased risk of heart disease and a 20-21% increase of getting type 2 diabetes for women and men respectively. One reason for this reduced risk for those having a good breakfast is because of what you eat in a typical meal, such as eating a cereal fortified with vitamins -- not the sugar type cereals that are especially designed for kids.

Another research study in the UK which investigated what 1600 young people ate for breakfast found that those who ate breakfast regularly had a better intake of fiber and micronutrients, including folate, vitamin C, iron, and calcium. Other studies in Australia, Brazil, Canada, and the United States found similar results.

Then, too, over 54 studies found that eating breakfast improves the functioning of your brain, most notably by improving your memory, and many studies show an improved ability to concentrate.[3]

Still other studies support eating a high-protein breakfast, because they reduce your craving for food later in the day, so you eat less, which contributes to your weight-loss, too.

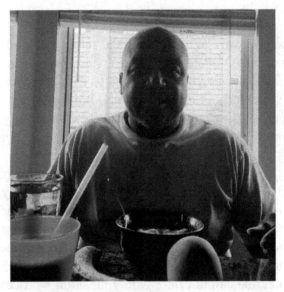

Yet, within these general guidelines for healthy eating, studies on what to eat show that there is no particular type of breakfast to eat. Thus, you can choose what you want to eat, as long as you follow the guidelines for good nutrition. Also, while it's a good idea to eat an early breakfast in light of the findings about the circadian rhythm, the research doesn't specify exactly when you should eat it. Rather, the research suggests listening to your body and eating when you are hungry, most notably when you wake up and feel hungry in the morning.

At the same time, your good breakfast should prepare the way for eating well throughout the day. This way you don't over-emphasize a single meal but eat well all day. As one expert on nutrition put it: "A balanced breakfast is really helpful, but getting regular meals throughout the day is more important to leave blood sugar stable through the day, (since) that helps control weight and hunger levels…Breakfast isn't the only meal we should be getting right."[4]

Understanding How Your Body Turns What You Eat Into Energy

In case you want to understand the science behind the way your body turns what you eat into energy, here's a brief overview, which will help convince you of the need to eat a good breakfast and have a healthy diet to both lose weight and build your strength.

As an article in *Better Health* describes, your body derives its energy from glucose. Besides getting that from the sugars you eat, glucose is broken down and absorbed into your body from the carbohydrates you eat. After that, your body stores most of this energy it produces as fat, and it stores some glucose as glycogen. It stores most of this glycogen in your liver, and smaller amounts go into your muscles. This glucose is especially important for your brain, which almost exclusively gain its energy from glucose.[5] So if your blood sugar drops down because you aren't getting enough glucose, that decline can interfere with your brain's processing, so you may not be as sharp as usual. You may not be able to concentrate or remember things as well.

A good reason for eating an early breakfast when you wake up in the morning from sleeping at night (or whenever you wake up later if you're on a shift schedule) is that you haven't eaten for 10 to 12 hours. During this time -- or if you fast for a while, your liver breaks down this glycogen and releases it as glucose to keep the level of your blood sugar stable, which is very important for your brain, which gets almost all of its energy from glucose. Then, once you eat breakfast, you add to the stores of energy and nutrients in your body.

In the event you run out of glucose fuel from glycogen because you haven't eaten for a while, your body goes to the next best thing -- the fats stored in your body. As the *Better Health* article explains, once your glycogen stores are used up, your body "breaks down fatty acids to produce the energy you need." But if you don't have carbohydrates to support this process, your body only partially oxidizes these fatty acids, which can reduce your energy level. By contrast, if you eat a good breakfast, that "boosts your energy levels and restores your glycogen levels," so they can keep up your metabolism for the day.[6] In fact, researchers have found that those who eat breakfast not only have more energy, but they tend to be more physically active in the morning than those who put off eating until later in the day.

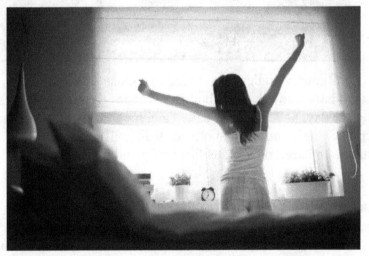

The research also shows that those who eat breakfast are more likely to meet a recommended daily intake of vitamins compared to those who don't do this. These key nutrients you get from common breakfast foods include folate calcium, iron, B vitamins, and fiber. Certainly, you can supplement the vitamins you get from food with store-bought bottles of multi-vitamins and individual vitamin and mineral supplements. However, according to scientists, many essential vitamins, minerals, and other nutrients can only be gained from food. Thus, even if your body can tap its stores of glycogen to get the glucose needed for energy until you eat again, you still need the vitamins and minerals from food to maintain your health and vitality.

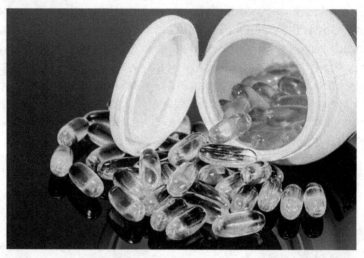

Still other studies have found that those eating an early breakfast have a lower BMI (body mass index), consume less fats during the day, have a higher daily calcium and fiber intake, and better meet the recommendations for fruit and vegetable consumption based on various factors, including their body weight.[7]

What Should You Eat for Breakfast?

You can eat a wide variety of food for breakfast; you don't need to eat a particular diet. What's important is that whatever you eat should be nutritious and healthy. Following are some suggestions, based on what I have chosen to eat myself and also recommended by various nutritionists.

1) <u>A porridge made from rolled oats</u>. If you make this from quick oats, select the plain variety and add your own fruit, rather than selecting a prepackaged porridge, since these tend to have a lot of extra sugar.

2) a wholegrain, high-fiber cereal, such as one made from bran, whole-wheat, or muesli; then you add in low-fat milk, soy or rice milk substitute, natural yogurt, and fresh fruit.

3) fresh fruits, such as sliced apples, pears, and pineapple; though avoid canned fruits in heavy syrup, since these are very high in sugar.

4) wholegrain, sourdough, high-fiber toast, English muffins, or bagel with a variety of healthy toppings, such as tomatoes, baked beans, poached or boiled eggs, mushrooms, spinach, salmon, cheese, avocado, hummus, or a 100% nut paste, such as made from peanut or almond butter.

5) smoothies made from nutritious ingredients, such as fresh fruit, vegetables, milk, and natural yogurt.

6) certain low-sugar and low-fats protein bars, combined with natural yogurt and a glass of low-fat milk or soy or rice milk substitute.

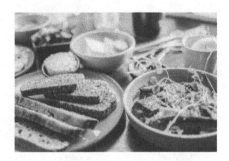 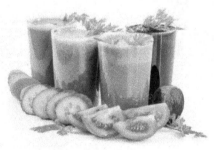

The goal of making these choices is that you want to select from these major food types to give you the sufficient nutrients and protect you from feeling hunger during the day. These four groups are the following, according to Molly Behan in "Benefits of Breakfast," writing for the University of New Hampshire Healthy UNH blog:

- Whole grains, obtained from cereals and oatmeal that are low in sugar and high in fiber, such as obtained from whole-wheat toast or half of a wheat bagel;

 - Lean protein, such as from peanut butter, hard-boiled eggs or lean meats;

 - Low-fat dairy, such as skim or low-fat milk, cottage cheese, and yogurt with a low amount of sugar;

 - Fruits and vegetables, fresh or frozen fruit, or 100% fruit juices with no added sugar. Smoothies full of fruits and vegetables are also fine.[8]

 When you purchase any processed breakfast foods, check the labels to make sure they are healthy and nutritious. Be especially careful with protein bars and some yogurts, since some of these have a lot of added sugar. Ideally, says Christy C. Tangney, a clinical dietician at Rush University Medical Center, it is best to "keep your sugars under 20 grams and look for bars with about 6 to ten grams of protein and three or more grams of fiber."[9]

CHAPTER 4: INCREASING YOUR STRENGTH THROUGH LIFTING WEIGHTS

Besides eating a good breakfast, eating other healthy nutritious meals, and reducing my calorie intake, I found lifting weights a critical additional activity. This is because the weight lifting contributed to my ability to do more exercise, such as walking, since it gave me more energy. It also improved my muscles, and my body became strong.

In this chapter I want to discuss in detail the many benefits of weight training and how you can lift weights to improve your own health, vitality, and strength.

The Benefits of Lifting Weights

There are a great many benefits of lifting weights, variously referred to as "weight training" "resistance training," or "strength training." The goal of this training is to improve your muscular fitness by exercising a specific muscle or muscle group against some type of external resistance. This resistance can be from free weights, such as barbells or weight machines, or you can use your own body weight, such as when you do pushups. The basic principle is that you apply a load or weight in order to put pressure on the muscle by overloading it, which makes it adapt and get stronger.

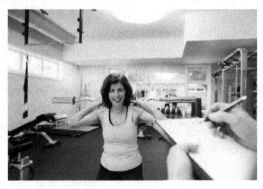

There are two types of resistance training:
- Isometric resistance, in which you contract your muscles against a nonmoving object, such as the floor, when you do a pushup.
- Isotonic strength training, in which you contract your muscles as you engage in a range of movements when you lift weights.

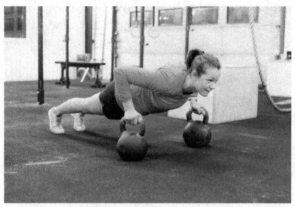

Here are the major benefits of weight training according to many fitness trainers and medical practitioners.

1) It makes you stronger and fitter. This benefit may seem obvious, since the purpose of lifting weights is to increase your muscle strength. Then, these stronger muscle increase your ability to participate in the activities of daily living, as well as to do physical work, They do so, because you have more muscular and bone strength, so you can work harder and longer. Plus you have more endurance. For example, when your legs get stronger, you can spend more time walking, exercising on a treadmill, or going on a hike. That benefit occurs for runners, too, since they can run more efficiently when they also lift weights. This is the case because when they run at the same speed, they use a lower capacity of their leg strength, as author Carmen Chai points out in an article: "8 Reasons Why Weight Training Is Incredible for Your Health."[10]

2) <u>It increases your bone density</u>. This increase in density is very important, especially as you get older, since the body tends to lose bone mass, and as you lose more, your bones can become brittle and more apt to break. The body loses that mass because it constantly absorbs and replaces bone tissue. However, as individuals age, they are increasingly prone to osteoporosis, a disease in which new bone creation doesn't keep up with old bone removal -- a condition that affects one out of three women and one out of five men over 50. Thus, women are particularly prone to bone loss in that they make up 80% of the cases of osteoporosis due to the loss of bone mass.[11] In fact, you may have this condition but not know it, since many people have no symptoms until they have a bone fracture, though a doctor may recognize a loss of bone mass when doing a bone density test during a physical. or those with this condition, treatment includes medications, such as Alendendronate Sodium, eating a healthy diet, and exercising with weights to help prevent bone loss or strengthen already weak bones.

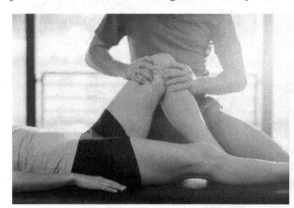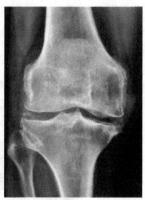

3)<u> It increases the strength of your connective tissue, muscles, and tendons</u>. By increasing this strength, not only do your bones become stronger, but so do all of your connective tissues which are used to move your bones. As a result, due to improved motor performance, you can move better, and you are less likely to sustain any injuries.

This increased strength occurs, since <u>weight training</u> <u>promotes a lean, fat-free muscle mass, which decreases with age</u>. This decrease in muscle mass starts at around 30 years of age, when individuals lose up to 3 to 5 percent of this mass each year. Without strength training, your muscles, especially in your arms and legs, will turn into fat, and as this deterioration progresses, this reduction in mass can lead to "scarcopenia," a syndrome characterized by progressive and generalized loss of skeletal muscle mass and strength. Eventually, as this condition progresses, one can experience a physical disability, poor quality of life, and even death. While the risk factors include age, gender, and level of physical activity, you can decrease your chances of getting this syndrome by developing lean fat-free muscles through lifting weights. For example, a study published in the October 2017 issue of the *Journal of Bone and Mineral Research* reported that postmenopausal women with low bone mass increased their bone density, structure, and strength, as well as their functional performance, by spending just 30 minutes twice a week in high intensity resistance and impact training.[12]

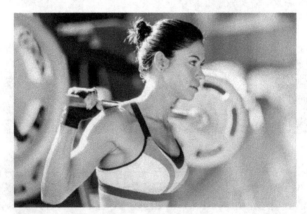

4) <u>It will help you develop your body mechanics by</u> <u>improving your balance, coordination, and posture</u>. That improvement in your body mechanics occurs because stronger

muscles help you have better balance, stand straighter, and coordinate your movements. One reason for your better balance is that many strength-training movements require balance and mobility from your body. As Lauren del Turco notes, as you move around in building your strength, you use different planes of motion and different angles, so your major muscle groups and smaller muscles become stronger and more stable.[13] This improved balance helps to prevent falls, too, as one study showed. It found that older people, who have a higher risk of falling due to poorer physical functioning, had a 40% lower risk of falling as a result of lifting weights.

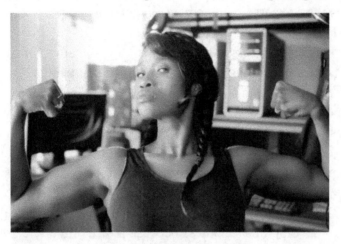

5) <u>It increases your metabolism and fat loss</u>. This occurs because you burn more calories if you have more muscle. A muscle burns more calories compared to fat, because it is an active tissue, so even when you are at rest, it burns more energy. A way to think of this process is to compare it to what happens with a thermostat in your house. Say your body is like that house. When you engage in an aerobic exercise, that exercise raises the heat for about 30 to 40 minutes while you work out. By contrast, when you engage in strength training, that doesn't turn up the heat as much, but the burn lasts for a longer time.[14]

6) It helps you keep the weight off for good, and you will burn more calories during the day, because you have more muscles and less fat. Weight training contributes to this result, because your body has to burn more calories to maintain muscle compared to fat. weight training can increase your metabolism so you burn more calories. This training also supplements the weight loss you gain as a result of aerobic exercises, such as walking, running and cycling. A key reason for this greater weight loss, according to an article by doctor Chris Iliades, "7 Ways Strength Training Boosts Your Health and Fitness," in *Everyday Health*, is that a good resistance workout increases your excess post-exercise oxygen consumption, also called EPOC. Then, your body continues to burn calories after a workout, which "keeps your metabolism active after exercising, much longer than an aerobic workout." Researchers have documented this finding. For example, a study published in the *Obesity* journal in November 2017 found that the dieters who did strength training exercises four times a week for 18 months lost more fat (about 18 pounds) compared with the weight lost by non-exercises (who lost only 10 pounds) and the aerobic exercisers (who lost 16 pounds).[15]

7) It can transform your body, so you have a sleeker, leaner look. You develop this sleekness because if you only use cardio to change the amount of muscle versus fat on your frame, you will typically plateau quickly. But consistent strength training can transform your physique. As described by Laruen del Turco in a LiveStrong article: "11 Benefits of Strength Training that Will Convince You to Lift Weights," when you gain muscle and lose fat that will make your arm and legs look more defined. While cardio can help you lose weight, strength training gives you strong, defined shoulders.[16]

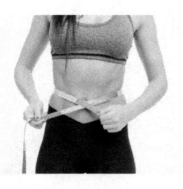 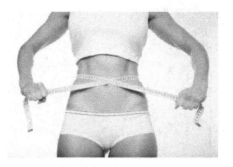

8) <u>It has cardiovascular health benefits</u>. These benefits to your heart health occur because strengthening your muscles helps to improve your blood pressure. According to the U.S. Health and Human Services Department's recommendation, you should do muscle strengthening activities two times a week plus engage in at least 150 minutes of weekly moderate-intensity activity to reduce hypertension and lower the risk of heart disease.

9) <u>It staves off disease and helps people with chronic diseases better manage them</u>. This occurs because strength training contributes to overall wellness. As researchers have found, strength training, along with cardio and other types of activity, reduce the chances of getting any of the chronic diseases, including cardiovascular disease and cancer. Additionally, strength training helps individuals with a chronic disease better manage the symptoms. For example, individuals with arthritis find that strength training can be as effective as taking medications to reduce their arthritis pain. This training also helps individuals with type 2 diabetes improve their glucose control -- a benefit for the 14 million Americans who suffer from this condition. [17] Strength training contributes to this improvement, because it helps burn through glucose, which keeps down your blood sugar level.

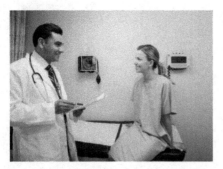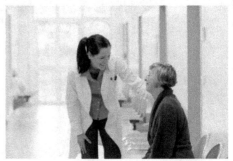

10) It reduces inflammation, which occurs with many diseases as well as injuries. While experts have found no clear reason why weight lifting helps with inflammation, a number of studies found that regular resistance training sessions about twice a week led to lower inflammation in overweight women. [18]

11) It helps you feel more energy and improves your mood. When you lift weights you will feel generally better, too. You will feel happier and more energetic. A key reason for this uplift in your spirits and energy is that strength training increases your level of endorphins, which are the natural opiates produced by the brain. These lift your energy levels and improve your mood, as do other exercises, as long as you exercise in an appropriate way, so you don't overly tire yourself.

12) It improves your overall quality of life and your confidence. This improvement occurs because you not only can do more things, but you feel more confident in your abilities. In turn, this greater assurance helps you better manage your weight, as well as gain more strength.[19] Another way this training increases your self-esteem and self-confidence is when you set a new personal best in the weights you lift, so you lift heavier weights or lift weights for a longer period of time, according to Dr. Stuart Phillips, a professor of kinesiology at McMaster University.[20] Then, as you achieve each

goal, you not only feel healthier, but you feel more confidence, because you have achieved that goal.

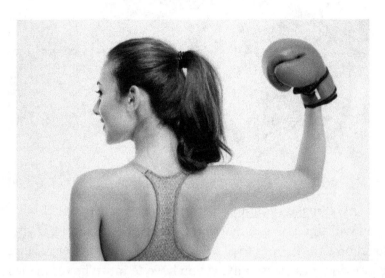

13) <u>It improves your mental health</u>. While extensive research has shown that aerobic or cardio exercises, such as walking and cycling, can improve your mental health, researchers are now finding that strength training is linked to better mental health, too. For example, according to Lauren del Turco, a July 2013 review in *Neuropsychobiology* found that "strength training, particularly high-intensity strength training, can help lessen symptoms in people with depression." Moreover, the researchers concluded that combining a moderate intensity aerobic training with high-intensity strength training provided more positive benefits than any other exercise programs.[21] Thus, a combination of both aerobic and strength training exercises is ideal, which is what I did -- I combined running for about 20 to 30 minutes each day with 20 to 30 minutes of lifting weights.

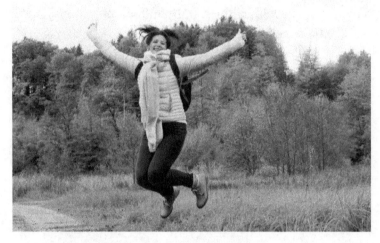

14) <u>It makes your everyday tasks easier</u>. No matter what you do, you will find you can more easily do it. For example, if you have to stand on your tip toes to reach something, your better balance will help you do this successfully. If you have to move boxes in cleaning out your house or preparing to move, you will have more strength to do this. If you work at a desk job and have to sit at a computer all day, your stabilizer muscles in your torso, which play a major role in your posture, will increase your endurance, so you can stay erect and not feel tired.[22]

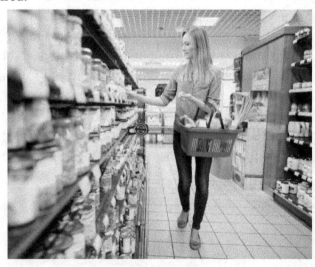

15) <u>It supplements the benefits you get from participating in aerobic exercises</u>. That's because weight training, like running or other aerobic exercises, is good for "your heart, your brain, your waistline, and your mental health," as Carmen Chai points out in a *Global News* article: "8 Reasons Why Weight Training Is Incredible for Your Health."[23]

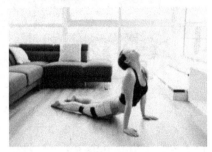 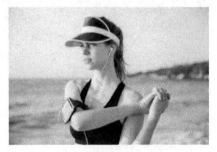

16) <u>It's good for your heart</u>. Even though cardio exercises have long been credited as being good for your heart, strength training contributes, too. For instance, in a study reported in the January 2017 *Medicine and Science in Sports and Exercise*, the researchers found that women who engaged in any strength training had a 17% lower risk of developing cardiovascular disease than those who did no strength training. [24]

17) <u>It can improve your performance in sports</u>. No matter what type of sports you participate in, strength training will help you do better. It will especially help you in sports that require a lot of short bursts of power or longer periods of low activity and rest, such as golf or tennis. It can help you run faster, too, as a number of research studies have shown. For instance, a 2016 study reported in the *Journal of Strength and Conditioning Research* found that professional soccer players who participated in six weeks of strength training had a much improved sprinting ability, and a 2014 study reported in the *Scandinavian Journal of Medicine and Science in*

Sports found that cyclists who participated in 25 weeks of heavy lifting were able to pedal more powerfully.[25]

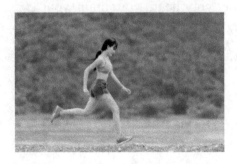 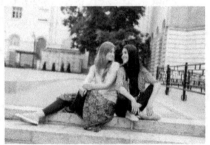

18) <u>It makes your routine more challenging and interesting</u>. It does so by adding variety to your workout. If you do the same cardio workouts again and again, you can find this gets boring. But when you engage in strength training, this can "spice things up and add a completely different challenge to your body," as Paige Waehner notes in "Why You Should Lift Weights and Strength Train" in a March 11, 2020 posting on *VeryWellFit*. As she points out, strength training offers many different ways to set up your workouts, so you can always try something new by adding new exercises, different types of resistance, new routines, and a variety of ways to work your body.[26]

19) <u>It can help you live longer</u>. Studies have found a link between strength, muscle mass, and longevity. A study at the University of Pittsburg of 70 to 79-year-old women found this link, when they learned that women with stronger quadriceps muscles (the large muscles at the front of your thigh) and stronger hand grips lived longer the stronger their muscles. The researchers found that it was the muscle strength, not their size, that made the difference.[27]

Getting Started with Your Own Weight Lifting Program

It is best to get some guidance when you first start lifting weights, rather than just running out and buying weights or finding objects at home you can lift, such as heavy cans or reams of paper. You might be able to use such objects as well as weights, but a fitness or physical training professional can help you make good decisions about setting up your weight lifting program. For example, they can help you decide what kind of equipment to use and how heavy the weights you lift should be. They can also help you determine how often and for how long you should lift weights in the beginning and as you continue in the program.

Thus, it's a good idea to set up an initial appointment with a personal trainer or fitness specialist. They can show you how to lift the weights effectively, explain the basics of a successful strength training program, and set up a weekly program for you. They can also explain how you can gradually increase the weights and other exercises you do, so you keep on achieving additional strength and endurance. Or perhaps take a class, such as offered by your local physical therapy center or YMCA.

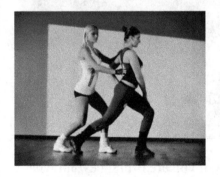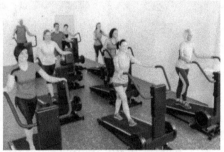

When you set up a program for yourself, keep in mind these basic principles.

1) Start slowly with smaller weights and a shorter program of lifting. Later you can increase the amount of weight you lift and the length of your activity. By taking it slow, you reduce your

chances of sustaining an injury or feeling really sore after your exercises.

2) Start with single sets of weights, and later you can add additional weights. For instance, a good starting level is lifting 5 pound weights for 5 minutes; then you might work yourself up to 8 or 10 pound weights for 8 to 10 minutes. Your trainer or fitness specialist can recommend the correct combination of weight levels and the amount of time for doing these lifts.

3) Use the correct weight amount -- not too little and not too much. If you don't lift enough weight, you won't provide your muscles a sufficient challenge, so you won't experience the benefits of weight training. Conversely, if you lift too much weight, you will increase your chances of being injured or becoming overly tired and drained of strength. A good way to know if you are lifting too much is that you will find it hard to lift the last repetitions of the exercise, because you feel less energy to go on.

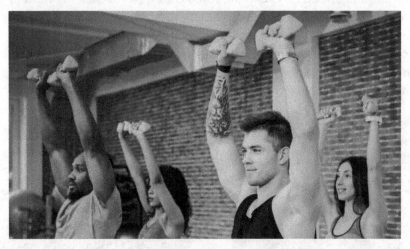

4) Gradually increase the weight you are lifting beyond what you think you can lift. You want to stay within safe limits, so don't try to lift weights you can barely pick up. But you can gradually lift heavier and heavier weights to build your strength.[28]

5) Figure on spending at least 20 to 30 minutes every other day, unless you want to do more. A good way to do a workout is

with three short sets -- 12 repetitions or reps per set. In each set include weights and combination of exercises to target all the major muscle groups, a recommendation from Len Center, a *Healthday* reporter for Medical Xpress.[29]

6) Allow your muscles in each muscle group time to rest and recover. Generally, you should wait at least 48 hours before you exercise those same muscles again.

7) If you feel bored doing the same exercise routine, you can vary your routine to keep this training from becoming boring. For example, you can add variety to your routine by variously using machines, free weights, bar bells, kettlebells, and bars as you train. You can also switch up the number of sets, the time between sets, your choice of different exercises, and varying your speed. You might also put on some music to listen to as you exercise -- either through a player in the room or listen to the music through headphones.

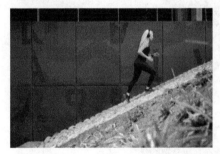 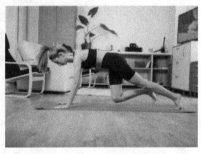

8) If you don't have any gym equipment to train with, you can lift some heavy objects around your house or office. To this end, you can use some heavy cans, some sacks of flour, even a ream or two of paper. The idea is to look around your house and see what you have that is heavy; then practice with that. As you become comfortable lifting objects that weigh a certain amount, you can add others to increase the weight.

9) If you are new to strength training, a good way to do this safely and effectively is to first get an okay from a doctor; then work with a trainer on the best type of training for you.

10) For variety, you might combine your strength training at home with some recordings of things you want to learn or enjoy. For example, put on an audiobook and listen as you train. The audiobook might be a how-to book about something you want to learn, a bestseller to keep you informed, or a chapter from a novel you find entertaining or exciting.

11) Think of your workout as a kind of meditation, so you can combine it with mindfulness exercises, soft music to relax, or ask yourself questions and let your unconscious give you the answers as you practice.

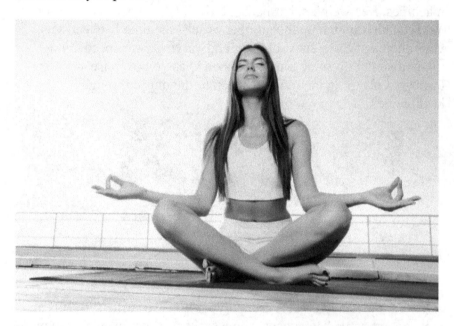

CHAPTER 5: UNDERSTANDING HOW YOUR BODY BURNS CALORIES TO SHAPE YOUR DIET

It is helpful to know how your body burns calories, so you can better choose a good healthy diet and do a better workout to build your strength. Accordingly, I'll describe the basic process of burning calories here.

The body's two basic fuels are glucose, which is stored as glycogen, and fat. Importantly, glucose and glycogen are anaerobic fuels, so they can provide energy without oxygen, whereas fat is an aerobic fuel, so oxygen must be present to burn it. As Ed Blonz points out in "How the Body Burns Fuel During Exercise," our muscles are "primed to burn fat" which is "our most concentrated form of energy."[30] When we start to exercise, we initially burn glucose and glycogen, but within minutes, the body begins burning fat. It is a smooth transition, and the more fit your body, the smoother this transition.

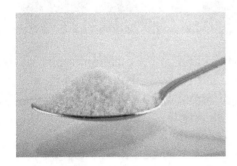 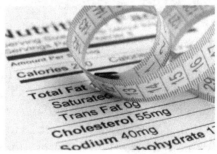

As Blonz explains, when we are resting, only a very small amount of fats are in the bloodstream, and our breathing and heartbeat are relaxed, so we take in just enough oxygen and pump blood at a slower rate sufficient for our needs at the time. But once you start to exercise, your muscles respond immediately. Your heart starts to beat faster and your breathing becomes deeper. Should you be out of shape and push too hard, you will soon feel out of breath and have to stop. But if you are in shape, you can push harder without becoming tired and out of breath.

The reason for this reaction is the way your body burns glucose, glycogen, and fats. Initially, the body gets its energy from glucose and glycogen. At the same time, the brain sends a signal to the areas which store fat to send some fuel. It also signals the lungs to begin breathing more quickly to provide more oxygen and begin removing carbon dioxide, which is released as your muscles begin working.

How Your Body Burns Carbs, Proteins, and Fats

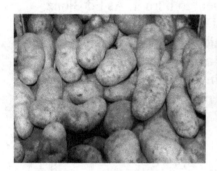 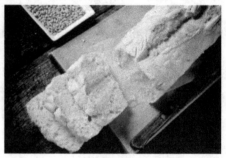

More specifically, your body obtains three different types of fuel -- carbohydrates or sugars, fats, and proteins, but it burns them at different times, rates, and under different circumstances, as described in a *VirtualMedStudent.com* article: "Understanding Carbs, Proteins, and Fats and How the Body Burns Them."[31] The carbohydrates, called "carbs" for short, are burned first. They are composed of sugar molecules that are linked together in various arrangements. The most important carbohydrate is starch, which is composed of numerous glucose molecules linked together in a long strand. Some common types of starches are potatoes and bread.

Another type of carbohydrate is glycogen, which is the way we store excess glucose for later use. But instead of being composed of a long strand of individual glucose molecules, as in starch, glycogen is composed of many branches, so the body can readily pull off individual sugar molecules to be burned for energy. There are two types of carbs -- simple and complex carbohydrates. The simple carbs are made up of a few sugar molecules linked together, generally one to three of them, while the complex carbs are made up of multiple sugar molecules linked together in a complicated way.

A key difference during digestion is that simple carbs are quickly absorbed in the stomach and enter the blood stream very quickly, such as when you eat a candy bar, which gives you a quick boost of energy. But because they enter the bloodstream quickly, your body metabolizes them rapidly, so after you get a quick energy boost, you quickly feel de-energized after about an hour.

By contrast, complex carbs are absorbed much more slowly, so you get a more continuing but less intense energy boost. A good example of complex carbs is the whole grains in whole wheat bread or oatmeal.

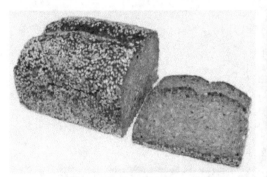 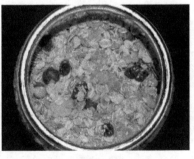

When you exercise, the glucose or glycogen in carbs is the first energy source your body uses. This is one reason that some fitness trainers recommend carb loading, whereby you eat a meal high in carbohydrates the night or morning before you work out. By doing so, when you exercise, your body will use the sugar molecules in the carbohydrates to give you energy for your muscles and brain.[32] Then, after your body uses up the carbs, your body will look to fat and protein for its other fuel sources.

The body burns fat next, because fat doesn't provide energy as efficiently as sugar. You can tell the moment when you burn up all your carbs and your body switches over to burning fat, since you will experience a sudden feeling of fatigue. That's because you are now getting less energy per unit of fat, compared to the greater energy you get per unit of glucose or glycogen. This experience is especially noticeable when you work your muscles too hard. In this case, your body uses up the available glucose before the fats and oxygen arrive, so your muscles run out of energy.

On the other hand, the more fit you are, the faster and more easily your body shifts from anaerobic to aerobic burning -- from burning glucose and glycogen to burning fats. Taking some time to warm up or start slowly will further help the burning process, because the brain will send out the signal earlier to start burning fat, and that will shift the blood flow to the working muscles. Yet, even after your body shifts to burning fats, it will continue to burn some glucose, which leads the muscles to produce lactic acid. This goes to the liver, which recycles that acid back into glucose.[33]

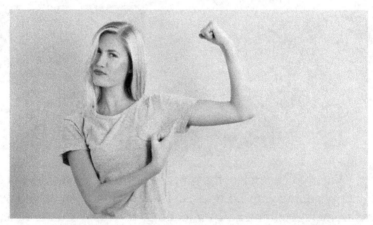

Thus, as you become more fit, you have more energy from your muscles, so you can exercise for a longer time and more effectively. But if you try to get your muscles to act more quickly or for a longer period than they can, you will experience what's called "hitting the wall" -- the feeling that you can't do anymore, because you are suddenly very exhausted. Your body has essentially run out of gas. Should you try to press on, your body will seek to burn more glucose to provide that extra energy. But eventually, that will lead your liver to produce even more lactic acid to fill the energy gap. Over time, this lactic acid will build up, so you will experience painful cramps and feel exhausted, and your muscles will no longer be able to work.[34]

As a result of this burning process, where glucose and fats burn first, these supply your body with initially short-term and then long-term energy. In fact, this burning process for glucose actually begins in your mouth through the action of your saliva. Even before you take your first bite, your saliva starts forming in your mouth, anticipating what you are going to eat. Once you start eating, the enzyme in your saliva called "amylase" starts the process of breaking down your carbs into simpler structure. When your food gets to your stomach, it is further broken down, and in the small intestine, the amylase secreted by the pancreas turns your carbs into simple sugars, which are absorbed into the bloodstream. Thereafter, these sugars are transported to the cells which use them for energy.[35]

However, the process is even more complicated than that, since there are different types of carbs which burn more or less quickly, as Jody Braverman points out in "Do Carbs or Protein Burn First." The simple carbohydrates like sugar burn most quickly, whereas complex carbs, such as starches, have a more complex molecular structure, so the body takes a longer time to break them down. But the body doesn't break down fiber, the third type of carb, at all. The fiber just moves through the digestive track with almost no changes. Instead, it adds bulk to the waste which helps to move it along to be execrated.[36]

The way your body first burns sugars and then fats also affects the way you lose weight. If you don't exercise long enough, even if you exercise very vigorously, you won't lose weight, because this quick exercise mainly burns up the carbohydrates stored in the liver as glycogen. But this burning doesn't touch the body's fat reserves.

The last type of fuel to burn is protein, which burns even more slowly. It comes from foods, such as beef, fish, nuts, and beans, and it has more complex structures derived from amino acids.

When your body breaks down protein, it separates the amino acids, which go to different parts of the body. Whereas the digestion process for carbs begins immediately in your mouth, your body doesn't start digesting proteins until the food reaches your stomach. There, a number of substances, including hydrochloric acid and a pepsin enzyme, break down the amino acids. Then, in the small intestines, more enzymes continue the digestion process by dissolving the proteins into amino acids. If you eat fatty proteins, such as fatty meats, that takes even longer to digest, since fats delay the emptying of your stomach into the small intestines.[37]

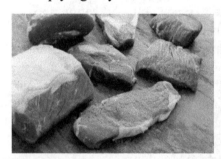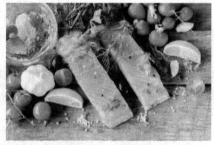

Generally, the body rarely burns protein, because it gets its energy from sugars and fats first. As a result, if you eat less than you should, your body starts starving itself when it burns off protein. In this case, the body uses the amino acid that underlies the creation of protein to form glucose in order to supply the brain with sufficient energy.

I observed a graphic example of what happens when the body goes into this starvation mode on the TV show *Alone.* In the sixth season, 10 contestants were placed by themselves in isolated sections of the Arctic. Once there, they had tents and some basic supplies for hunting and fishing. Then, they had to rely primarily on finding their own food in the form of fish, game, and a limited supply of vegetation, primarily blueberries. Over the course of 60 to 70 days for the longest lasting contestants, individuals wasted away, since they couldn't provide enough food for themselves. Several of them lost as much as 25-35% of their original body weight. As result of not getting enough food, towards the end, the contestants were very tired, sometimes disoriented. The producers even sent a few home, because they were in danger of their organs shutting down, and they could experience heart failure due to a lack of nutrition. Ironically, one of the contestants who had shot a moose, so he had plenty of protein, despite repeated thefts by local foxes and wolverines, was actually gradually starving his body. That's because the moose's body is made up largely of muscle, which is composed of protein, but it has very little fat, and the foxes and wolverines stole most of that. Though this contestant did outlast the others, who were in even worse shape, he ended up in a very low-energy weakened position, when he finally learned he had won and left for home at the end of the show.

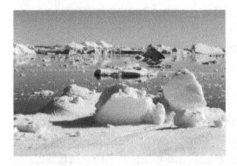 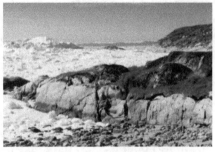

In short, your body first gets its energy from different types of carbohydrates. When it no longer has any glycogen stores to draw on, such as if you engage in a long-lasting and vigorous exercise or eat a very low-carb diet, your body will burn fat for energy. Then, if your body can't burn carbs or fats, it will turn to protein.[38] But that's like a last resort, so you want to keep your body fueled with carbs and fats, so you have enough to burn. This way you can exercise successfully, without depleting the proteins in your body.

Applying the Principles of How Your Body Burns Sugar, Fat, and Protein to Losing Weight

Given the way the body first burns sugars, fats, and finally protein, ISSA, the International Sports Sciences Association, which offers a certificate for fitness trainers, strength and conditioning coaches, and other health and medical professionals, offers some guidelines on the best way to burn fat, so you don't burn muscle. These guidelines include the following:

1) Recognize that the body is a "biogenetic continuum of energy systems" when you plan your workout. The fundamental unit of energy is adenosine triphosphate (ATP), which the body uses for fuel. The human body begins with enough ATP for 5 to 10 seconds of energy consumption before it begins to break down stored macronutrients to produce more ATP.[39] It starts with sugar, as previously described, since this is the easiest macronutrient to burn. So when you start to exercise for 10 seconds to several minutes, you primarily use glucose, drawing on the glycogen stored in your body. If you exercise intensely enough, your body will use glucose in the form of lactate. After several minutes, if you continue to exercise, your body will begin to burn fats to get its energy.[40]

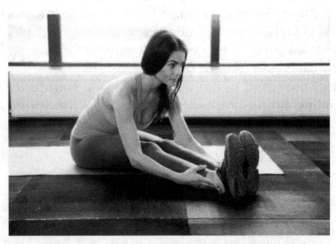

2) <u>Because of this burning process whereby the body burns calories by resynthesizing ATP, you will experience an excess post-exercise oxygen consumption (EPOC) effect</u>. This means that as the body burns calories, this process restores oxygen to your myoglobin, a protein, which carries and stores oxygen in the muscle cells and in your blood. Your body will also experience a higher core temperature and heart rate, and an increased respiratory rate. Additionally, you will experience a thermogenic effect, which is an enzymatic reaction that affects the basal metabolic rate. As your body's temperature heats up, so does your basal metabolic rate.

3) <u>When you engage in lower intensity and endurance workouts, which are aerobic activities, they first burn off the available sugar and then burn fat as fuel</u>. By contrast when you engage in anaerobic activities, which involve short exertion, high-intensity movements, such as in weight lifting, the main benefit comes after the exercise. That's because such activities break down glucose without using oxygen.

Based on these principles, you should fuel differently for your workouts on high-intensity and low-intensity days. It is best to alternate between high-intensity anaerobic exercises and low-intensity aerobic workouts to lose weight while gaining or not losing muscle. That means you should eat different types of foods for these days, as explained in the ISSA article "The Right Way to Burn Fat, Not Muscle."[41] Here's a breakdown on what you should do on different days.

1) <u>When Fueling for a Workout on High-Intensity Days</u>
These are the days when you are engaging in high-intensity workshops, such as lifting weights, especially heavier ones, for a longer time. On such days, low-carb fueling is not the most effective strategy, since your low glycogen level, which reflect your stored carbohydrates, combined with a high-intensity workout opens the door for burning the higher amounts of muscle, which you don't want to happen.

Accordingly, on a high intensity days, it is best to consume more protein, so you can rebuild your muscles. Additionally, eat carbs to make sure you have enough sugar to burn. A key reason for eating carbs on these days is, as the ISSA article explains, because eating carbs triggers the production of insulin, which is a powerful hormone that stimulates protein synthesis. Plus insulin releases blood sugar for energy use.[42] In this way, you can prevent your body from breaking down your muscle to burn protein to get energy.

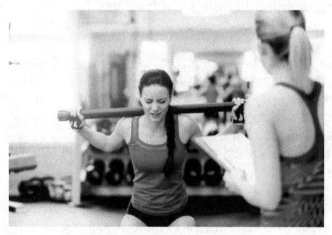

In short, ISSA recommends that you should consume complex carbs well before your workout and after it, because the body needs the insulin triggered by this process for protein synthesis after you finish working out.

2) When Fueling for a Workout on Low-Intensity Days
On low-intensity days, when you engage in aerobic workouts, your goal should be to burn fat, so everything you eat should be designed to trigger burning fat for energy, also known as "lipolysis." Accordingly, you should keep down your fat intake to less than 20% of your total calories, and you should keep down the level of carbs to less than 20% of your intake, since both are considered "enemies of lipolysis and fat burning."[43]

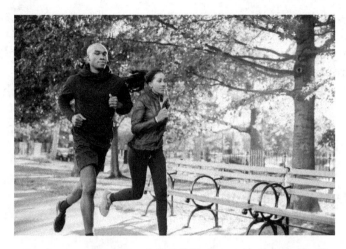

Another way to think of the difference between fueling your body on high-intensity and low-intensity days is to consider the role of lactate, which is a form of glucose your body uses during a high-intensity exercise. This lactate is used by the muscles for energy, or it is stored in the liver as glycogen. Since the body prefers to use glucose first for energy, the more lactate has accumulated in the body, the less fat you will burn during your aerobic low-intensity exercises. Since your high-intensity exercises result in a big increase in lactate production, you should avoid having this lactose build-up on low-intensity days, because you want to burn fat.

In other words, as ISSA notes, "the lower the exercise intensity, the higher the percentage of fat that is burned." By contrast, when you engage in higher aerobic intensity exercise, this not only causes fat to be burned, but it burns off a higher amount of your muscle.

Finally, pay attention to your heart rate, when you exercise on low-intensity days. Ideally, maintain your heart rate between 105 and 125 while you exercise.

3) The Advantage of Alternating High and Low-Intensity Days When Fueling Your Body

Given these different needs for fueling your body on high-intensity and low-intensity exercise days, in order to lose weight while you gain or avoid losing muscle, alternate your workouts and

73

your nutrition for high-intensity anaerobic exercise and low-intensity aerobic workouts. This means you should do the following to appropriately fuel your body.[44]

    - On high-intensity days, eat more and include carbohydrates in order to preserve muscle.

    - On low-intensity days, avoid carbohydrates and especially simple carbs in order to burn fat without losing muscle.

The Difficulty of Following this Approach to Appropriately Fuel Your Body

This approach recommended by ISSA may seem overly complicated and hard to follow. In fact, ISSA points out that it is both difficult and time-consuming to burn fat and maintain muscle. But don't seek a quick fix. Instead, consider varying your high-intensity and low-intensity diet. This is a slow but proven approach to successfully combine losing weight and building muscle.

Therefore, avoid diets that recommend drastically restricting your calories or cleaning your body. Initially, these low-calorie strategies combined with intense exercises can lead to immediate drops in your weight and clothing size. But they can create negative long-term effects on your health. That's why, ISSA emphasizes that you should "always focus on the long, slow, disciplined, and healthy approach to exercise and fueling."[45]

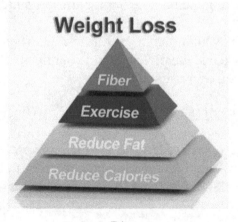

74

I kept these principles in mind when I did in my own exercise program, where I combined eating good healthy meals with running as an aerobic exercise and lifting weights an anaerobic exercise. Additionally, I started with a healthy nutritious breakfast.

I know it can be difficult to keep track of the different exercises you are doing and the different types of foods you are eating to alternate this low-intensity and high intensity approach to exercise and eating. Thus, I recommend creating a spreadsheet, such as on Excel, to map out your program and what you will do to exercise and eat on different days. You can also use this schedule to map your results, such as by noting your weight, waist size, and other measurements once a week or once a month. This way you can see very clearly how you are doing, and that can help motivate you to keep going, as you see the results you want.

CHAPTER 6: USING MEDITATION TO FURTHER YOUR PROGRESS

Meditation can also help you further your progress in losing weight, whether you already meditate or are just starting to do this. I started meditating in 2016, and this became an important part of my life, resulting in enormous differences. Meditation helped me center myself and get grounded. It also helped me let go of the past and forgive those in my life who did wrong to me, even back in my early childhood, such as the neighbor who molested me. I found this forgiveness through meditation very freeing. Additionally, meditation helped me feel more at peace with myself and with others. Though I sometimes have difficult days when I face various challenges or conflicts, as we all do, I feel I can better deal with these situations and make better choices. That's because meditation can give me answers to questions and provide me with more clarity in knowing where to go next.

Likewise, meditation can help you when you seek to lose weight, become more fit, and eat a healthier, more nutritious diet. Here are some ways it can help. Then, I will describe how to create and implement your own meditation program.

How Meditation Can Help Your Progress

Meditation can help your efforts to reduce your weight, eat better, and become stronger and fitter in these ways:

1) It can help you visualize yourself as you want to be. Then, what you visualize will help you set the goals you want to achieve.
2) It can help you visualize the different steps to take on the way to reach your goal.

3) <u>It can help you feel more relaxed and comfortable, when you participate in exercises or eat any meals during the day</u>. By feeling more relaxed and comfortable, you will more easily exercise, and you will have better digestion, so you can better burn calories, which will help you lose weight.

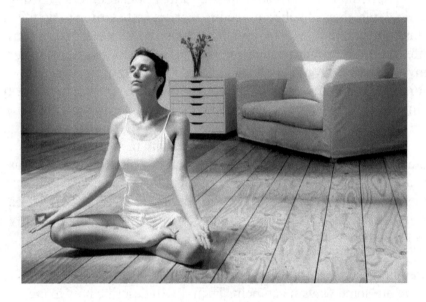

4) <u>It can help you better concentrate on what you are doing by shutting out any distracting thoughts</u>. This way you can better focus, and if you have any disrupting thoughts from your day, you can turn them off.

5) <u>It can quiet your mind, so you feel more peaceful and happier, when you exercise or enjoy a meal</u>.

6) <u>It can be combined with your exercises or with eating a meal</u>. This way, you remain in a meditative state during your exercises or your meals, if you participate in these activities alone.

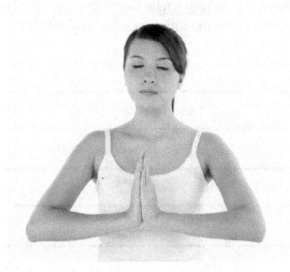

7) <u>It can contribute to a sense of community, if you meditate in a group with others who are pursuing a similar program</u>. In this case, you might set up a group meditation before you start on a walk, lift weights, or have a healthy, nutritious meal together.

8) <u>It helps you recognize and honor your achievements, as you meet certain goals and timelines along the way</u>. For example, you can visualize the reward at the end of achieving any goal you set for yourself, such as losing 5 pounds or lifting 10 pound weights. Then, when you have achieved that goal, you can experience receiving that reward in your mind as you meditate, and you will feel better and more committed to staying in the program.

9) <u>It can increase your commitment and determination, when you see yourself participating the activities you have set for yourself and then see yourself achieve your goal</u>.

10) <u>How else can meditation help to further your progress</u>?
Take some time to write down the different ways meditation can
help you.

_____

_____

_____

_____

_____

_____

_____

_____

_____

_____

_____

Different Ways to Meditate

There are many meditation methods, from chanting and Buddhist practices to mindfulness and focusing on eliminating all thoughts from your mind. Other meditative practices combine chanting and jumping around. Still others involve saying a special word, such as "ohm" again and again, as you sit in a lotus position with your eyes closed. Sometimes meditation occurs in a large group; other times you may meditate in solitude. Meditation can also occur in numerous settings, from your home to meadows and wooded groves in nature. Additionally, some meditation practices occur in silence or with soft meditative music in the background.

While some people are wedded to a particular meditation practice, others use different approaches. The times people spend in meditation vary, too -- from about 20 minutes every day or two to an hour or two each day. And sometimes individuals go to meditation retreats, where they spend a day or two, a whole weekend, or a week or more in meditation.

If you already have a meditation method that you use and like, you can continue to use that or use any of the suggestions here for meditating successfully. The following techniques can be combined with any traditional meditation practice or used to create your own method.

These techniques are based on those I used when learning how to do Mindful Meditation. This is an ideal way to gain more focus, reduce your stress, and inspire your creativity. It can take some time and practice to do a Mindful Meditation correctly, but you can easily learn the basics for how to do it. Once you learn this method, you can combine mindfulness techniques with whatever you do every day, such as when you are eating, going on a walk, exercising, or performing other daily tasks.

The basic way Mindful Meditation works is that you should take a break in your everyday routine. Then, pay attention to your surroundings. Next take a deep breath and feel your lungs expand. Now think about how you feel, but do so without any judgment. Just

81

acknowledge how you are feeling in the present and accept whatever those feelings are.

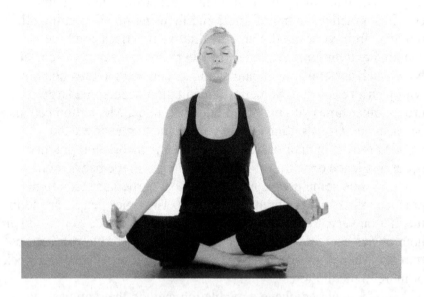

This approach has many similarities to but is different from some other common meditation methods, which include the following:

- In a guided meditation, you are led by a teacher, guide, or recording, where you go on a journey to a place you find calming and relaxing. Then, you visualize your surroundings and try to incorporate as many senses as you can, such as what you see, hear, smell, and touch.

- In a mantra or transcendental meditation, you select a word or phrase you feel is relaxing or calming. Then, you repeat it silently again and again to yourself. As you do, you seek to prevent any distracting thoughts from intruding on your thoughts. You shift your attention from these thoughts back to the calming word or phrase you are repeating.

- In a yoga or tai chi meditation, you breathe deeply as you engage in a slow series of different posture. As you move into these different postures, you focus on these movements rather than any stress you are experiencing in everyday life. Commonly, you need to take a class to learn the basic positions, and after that you can engage in these activities on your own.

- In deep breathing, you breathe deeply from your diaphragm, rather than taking the usual short shallow breaths from your chest. You continue this type of breathing until you feel calm and relaxed.

- In combining exercise with meditation, you go for a walk, run, or participate in another type of exercise, such as lifting weights, to clear your mind and feel more peaceful, relaxed, and get rid of any feelings of stress.

- In prayer, you use your own words or read prayers written by others. Then, you reflect on what these words mean to you or write down your thoughts in a journal.

You can use any methods that work for you, and you can combine them with Mindful Meditation, which is the primary method I use. Now let me tell you about the Mindful Meditation techniques I use and how to do it yourself.

Using Mindful Meditation

A good way to start Mindful Meditation is using a simple visualization exercise, where you see yourself in a comfortable safe space. You can imagine yourself in any place that feels safe for you. It can be a place where you have been before, either physically or in your imagination, or it can be a place that you have only seen, such as a picture in a magazine, book, or video. Alternatively, it can be a place you see for the first time in your imagination.

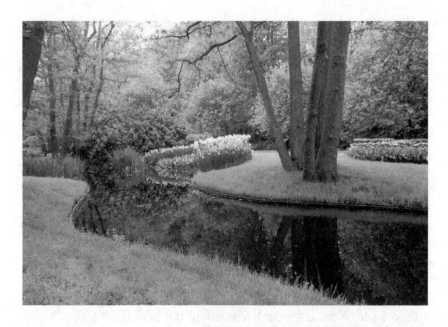

Wherever you do the meditation, get physically comfortable and go to a quiet place where nothing will disturb you, including any people around you or outside sounds. Then, sit in a comfortable position. While you can sit without any back to lean against, such as a cushion, ideally sit with your back against a chair and your feet firmly on the floor. Place your hands so they rest comfortably on your lap. Now you are not only in a safe space but in a safe position for the exercise.

Though you can visualize yourself in any place, a common visualization is to see yourself in a beautiful forest grove, where you are alone and all is peaceful. I'll give you an example about how you might create such a visualization in your mind. You can adapt your visualization to see yourself anywhere, such as on a mountain top gazing at the rolling hills and valleys around you, or on a beach watching the ocean waves go in and out calmly on a bright sunny day.

Here's how this visualization might go.

You are sitting on a log in a peaceful, beautiful forest. Look around, and visualize what this forest looks like. As you look up, you see a blue sky without any clouds -- or perhaps you see the golden and pink glow of a sunrise or sunset. Now look around you and notice the trees or grass. You notice the colors of the bark and leaves. Perhaps you see flowers around the trees. Then, you might notice a small stream or creek near you in the forest. You hear the stream or creek splashing over some rocks. Then, you hear the chirps of birds in the distance, and that reassures you that this forest is very peaceful and safe.

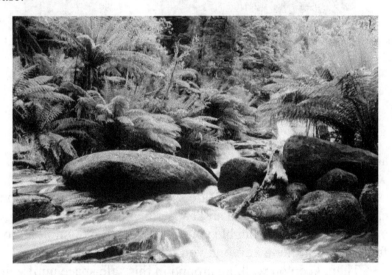

Meanwhile, continue breathing deeply and notice your breath going in and out, in and out. Then, you notice the smells around you, and you smell the scent of pine trees, wildflowers, and grass from a nearby meadow. As you breathe in these scenes, you feel a growing sense of peace and tranquility.

Now, in your imagination, you start walking to explore the forest grove and what's around it. You notice what's around you as you walk. You see clusters of trees, different kinds of flowers, rocks and boulders on the ground. Perhaps you see a few squirrels in the trees or scurrying along the ground.

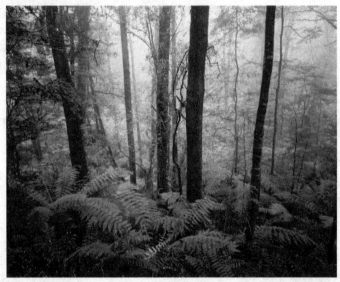

Then, in the distance, you might notice a small cottage, and perhaps you see a hammock between two trees there where you can rest. You can go there and relax if you want. As you relax, you feel your safe space all around you, and you can feel all your fears and anxieties going away, disappearing out of the safe space bubble you are in. You see them floating farther and farther away, and you feel totally at peace.

Then, keep on walking around in this safe space until you have viewed as much of it as you want. After that, return back to the grove where you started or to any place where you have walked that makes you feel very calm and peaceful.

Now as you see yourself sitting in this place, focus on your breathing. As you do, experience yourself feeling very peaceful and safe. Then, breathe in this way:

Inhale for a count of 1, 2, and 3; exhale for a count of 1, 2, 3. As you inhale and exhale, think to yourself, "I am very peaceful and safe."

Then, inhale again for a count of 1, 2, 3; and exhale for a count of 1, 2, 3. As you do, think to yourself, "I can always come to this safe peaceful space, when I am feeling fearful or anxious or if I feel overwhelmed by the stress in my life.

Now again inhale for a count of 1, 2, 3, and exhale for a count of 1, 2, 3. As you do, think to yourself: "This safe space will be here for me whenever I need it. I just need to know it's there, and I can go visit it again."

Finally, inhale for the last time for a count of 1, 2, 3, 4, 5, 6, and exhale for a count of 1, 2, 3, 4, 5, 6. As you do, tell yourself it is time to leave and return to the everyday world.

You can now open your eyes and come back into the room. Or if you need to, count backwards from 5 to 1, as you come back to everyday reality, feeling very calm, relaxed, and perfectly safe.

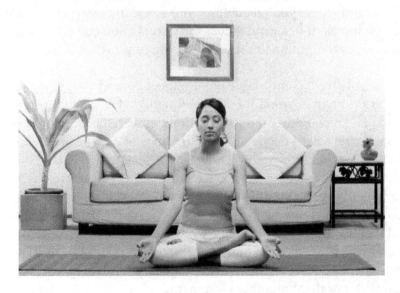

After you return from the meditation, continue to hold onto those feelings that you are very peaceful and perfectly safe, as you go about your daily activities.

Getting Set Up to Meditate

You want to create a good setting in which to meditate. Here are more specifics on how to select this place.

1) <u>You want a place where you won't have any distractions or interruptions</u>. This place can be a quiet room in your house, such as your own room, basement, or den, or someplace in your backyard, such as under a large tree. A very quiet section of a park is fine, too. Whatever place you choose, it should feel peaceful and enable you to separate yourself from the outside world.

If you are going to practice this meditation on a regular basis, you might create a special place that you use just for meditating. It doesn't have to be a whole room; it can be a special place within that room. For instance, you can set up a table at one side or in a corner of the room where you place items you find calming or inspirational, such as photos of beautiful places or flowers. You can also set up a few candles to light up this area when you turn off the lights.

2) <u>Have a comfortable environment around you, since you will be sitting in position for several minutes each time you meditate</u>. Among other things, the room temperature should be comfortable, and as needed, put the thermostat on a desired setting or adjust any heating or air conditioning. Also, as needed, sit on some pillows or cushions, or on a comfortable chair or couch. Additionally, since your body temperature may drop as you meditate, place some blankets around or near you. Then, you can start the meditation with a blanket wrapped around you or put it around you while you meditate. Alternatively, instead of using a room in your house, you can use a quiet, comfortable setting in a local park or other natural environment.

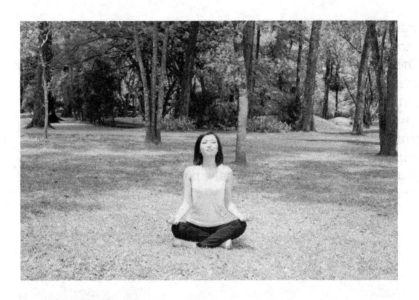

3) <u>Establish some time when you are going to meditate</u>.
When you first start meditating, 5 to 10 minutes can be a good way
to get comfortable with what you are doing. Later, you can spend a
little more time, say up to 15 to 30 minutes, much like you might
work yourself up to exercising for a short time and increase the time,
as you become more comfortable with the process. It's best not to
start with a long time initially, such as 45 minutes to an hour, since
spending this long in silence with only your thoughts can become
boring, and you can find yourself easily distracted. Instead start slow
and increase your meditation time by increments.

Since you may not be sure of the time and may want to
check it as you meditate, don't open your eyes to do this time check,
since this will break your focus and may stop the calming, relaxing
effect of meditation. Instead, it is better to use a timer with a soft
alarm that has a low hum or the sound of soft chimes, piano music,
or a gentle instrumental. This way you don't have to check the
timing, and the timer will bring you back in a soothing, gentle way.

4) <u>Experiment with different posture, because you can
meditate in any number of ways</u>. While sitting is common, you can
sit in any number of positions or places, not just in the legs-crossed

lotus position that is often associated with meditation. You can variously sit on a chair, couch, or the floor, and other positions are fine, too, such as if you want to stand or walk while you meditate. Lying down is also fine and very comfortable, but you have to be careful not to fall asleep and even start dreaming. If you do lie down, you might occasionally tap on the ground around you to remind yourself to stay awake. Feel free to try out different positions using cushions, pillows, or blankets, so you can find the position you like best -- or perhaps vary the positions you use at different times for variety.

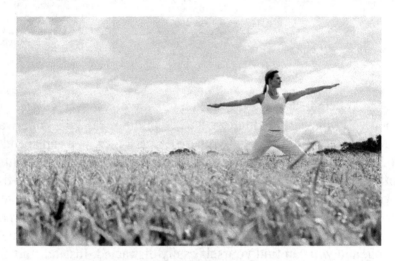

Having a Mindful Meditation

Now that you have set up your location and time for meditation and have gotten comfortable with whatever posture you are using, you are ready to start meditating. Here are the basic steps to follow:

1) <u>Relax and focus your mind, so you get settled; then begin to refocus your attention away from whatever is happening in your life</u>. It might take you a few minutes to relax and focus, and if your mind wanders back to your day to day activities, remind yourself to

focus on meditating again. For example, if you feel stress due to what happened during the day, you might find yourself reviewing and processing what happened. You may feel variously happy, sad, angry, regretful, or experience other emotions. Such feelings are very natural, since you bring to the meditation whatever happened during your day. Thus, you may need a few minutes to let your mind think about this. Then, too, if you are just starting to meditate, you may find that this mindful concentration feels unusual or strange, so you may need a few minutes to think about how you feel. The process is a little bit like releasing or letting go of your feelings of stress or other emotional feelings. You might even visualize these negative feelings going away, like they are flying out of the protective bubble around you as you meditate. However, you want to get relaxed, let any thoughts and feelings of the day bubble around in your mind. Then, as you get more and more relaxed, shift your consciousness to your physical position in the here and now. If necessary, shift your position around, so you are as comfortable as possible.

2) <u>Now focus on your breathing by taking some deep breaths</u>. As you turn your attention to your breath, pay attention to the way you are inhaling and exhaling with each breath. Experience your breath flowing in and out of your body as you inhale and exhale. Notice how your breath fills up your lungs and how you release it through your throat and mouth. After you observe this natural process for a minute or so, focus on breathing each breath more deeply and for a longer time. A reason for breathing more deeply is this will help your mind and body become calmer and more relaxed. In fact, just observing your breathing is a type of mindful practice, and if you want, you can devote a meditation to just observing your breathing going in and out. You will find this very calming, as I have experienced myself.

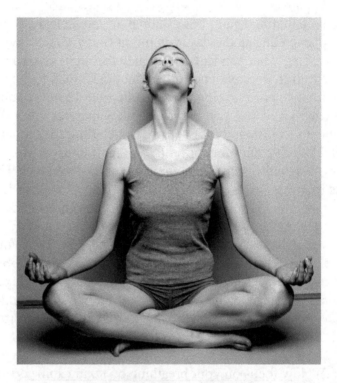

3) <u>Remind yourself that you are in control of your thoughts and emotions, because you are not your thoughts or feelings</u>. Having this control means you can choose what you want to pay attention to as you meditate. As a result, should you experience any thoughts or emotions that you don't want to engage with, you can send them away and shift your focus to what you want to think about and how you feel very calm and relaxed. Having this control also means you can transform any negative thoughts into positive ones or send them away. When you first start meditating, this transformation and letting go process may be unfamiliar to you. So don't be concerned if it takes time to easily shift your attention. Don't blame yourself if you can't do this right away. Remind yourself that you can do it, and practice sending away and letting go any negative thoughts or feelings. Keep on shifting your attention to what makes you feel calm and relaxed, and eventually those negative thoughts and feelings will go away.

4) <u>Keep returning your attention to your breathing whenever you experience any distractions</u>. You might experience these distractions from outside sounds, voices from another room, thoughts about the day, memories of something in your past, or anything else that interrupts your focus. If you do get distracted, a good way to get back to your meditation is to return to observing your breathing going in and out. Likewise, should any negative thoughts or feelings pop up, pay attention to your breathing again to get back on track. If you experience any negative thoughts or feelings, don't judge them or criticize the way you are meditating. You don't want to judge yourself in any way, because this judgment will disrupt your meditation experience, too. For example, don't tell yourself you are doing something wrong, because you suddenly thought of things that happened during the day or at another time in your life. This mental wandering is common, and when it happens, just return to your breathing and let such thoughts go.

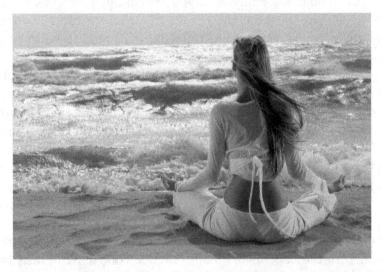

5) <u>Stay in the present and stop your mind from jumping back into the past or ahead to the future</u>. his emphasis on remaining in the present is a key goal of practicing a Mindful Meditation. Therefore, just as you want to return to your breathing if there are any distractions, you want to keep out any thoughts about what

happened in the past or what might happen in the future. If you have such thoughts, shift your attention back to your body, and especially to your breathing going in and out. This refocusing to stay concentrated on your meditation will help you remain centered and grounded in the present, and this present focus will help you feel calm and relaxed.

Practicing Mindfulness Everyday

Aside from engaging in specific mindful meditations each day, it helps to apply a mindful approach in your everyday life, including when you exercise. You can do this in at least four ways, and you may find other methods to help you live this mindful life.

1) <u>You can engage in mindful eating</u>. The idea here is to eat slowly, so you really enjoy what you are eating. When you eat more slowly, you pay more attention to the food you are eating, so you are more aware of the taste, smell, and feel of different foods in your mouth.

For example, you might do the following with a piece of fruit, such as an apple, banana, or pear, or with a vegetable, such as a carrot or tomato. A good way to start is with your sense of sight by looking closely at whatever you are holding. As you look, observe the food's shape, texture, and color. Next, to engage your sense of touch, feel the fruit or vegetable as you hold it in your hands or press it against your lips. Third, use your sense of smell by bringing the fruit or vegetable close to your face, and as you breathe in, notice how it smells. Also, notice any response from your body. For instance, your saliva may start to flow, and you increasingly want to taste the fruit or vegetable. Finally, engage your sense of taste by biting the fruit or vegetable and paying attention to the way it tastes, how it feels in your mouth, and how you like chewing it. While you can't take the time to engage in such an exercise for everything you eat, try doing this from time to time, and that will increase your enjoyment of food as you eat. The exercise will also help you be more attentive to other things in your life.

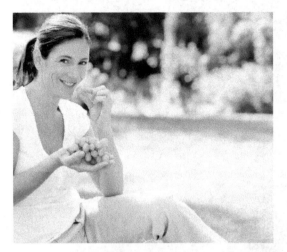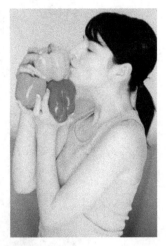

    2) <u>Participate in mindful walking</u>. Besides meditating in a sitting position, you can combine meditation with walking or participating in other exercises. The way to do this is to pay more attention to what you are doing as you walk or exercise. In particular, notice your feelings or emotions, and feel how your muscles respond as you move them. Notice any differences when you flex or stretch them. Then, as you walk or exercise, try slowing down, speeding up, and slowing down again, and pay attention to the differences. When you slow your movements, you may find you can pay even more attention to how you move and the sensations you feel, as you lift your feet up and then touch the ground, or as you raise and lower your arms while lifting weights. One way to feel even more sensations when you walk is to take off your shoes so you walk barefoot. That will help you feel more sensations, such as how the ground feels under your feet. You can notice how soft or hard or how warm or cool it is. Likewise, when you lift weights, you might notice the environment around you, such as the room temperature and if there is any breeze blowing as you work out. You can combine this close observation of your environment with yoga exercises, too.

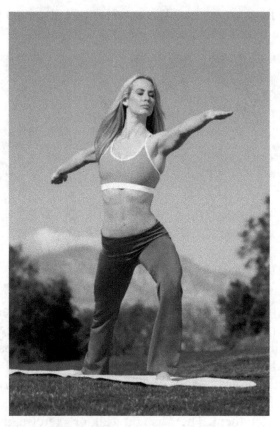

3) <u>Pay attention to the sensations in your body</u>. You can do this anytime to take a temperature check of how your body is feeling. It is especially helpful to pay attention to any sensations of pain or tension, since you can use this awareness to reduce your pain or tension. To get started, select a part of your body to pay attention to. This can be external, such as if you focus on your arms, legs, or face; or it can be internal, such as if you focus on how your heart is pumping or how your stomach feels. Then, ask yourself a series of questions about what you are experiencing. For instance, ask yourself if your sensations in that part of your body feel good, unpleasant, or neutral. Notice if you have any sensations of pain, and if so, you might rate this pain on a scale of 1-10. Then, you might imagine that the pain is going away; perhaps imagine yourself

96

sending healing energy to that spot. Soon you are likely to experience that pain subsiding or going away completely, and that part of your body might soon feel good. Notice the way your mind can influence how your body feels, and the way your body can affect the perceptions and thoughts in your mind.

One way to pay attention to your sensations in your body is to do a body scan. This way you shift your focus up and down your body, so you focus on the sensations in each part in turn. You might also notice how the energy flows up and down your body. This process is a little like a breathing and calming exercise in which you relax by shifting your attention to different parts of your body getting more and more relaxed, such as when you think this or a meditation leader tells you: "Now focus on your feet becoming more and more relaxed….Now your legs are becoming more and more relaxed….Now your stomach and chest are becoming more and more relaxed…Now your arms…" And so on.

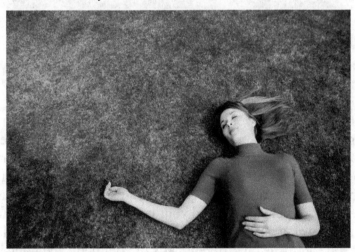

Another way to do this sensation exercise is to become more aware of each of your senses in turn. First, use your sense of sight to open your eyes and look around you. As you do, notice any objects or colors; be aware of any movements. Next, use your sense of smell to notice any smells in the air around you. Then, use your sense of hearing to listen for any sounds around you. For instance, do you hear any birds chirping; do you hear any traffic or voices of people outside; are there any background sounds in your house, such as of water or electricity?

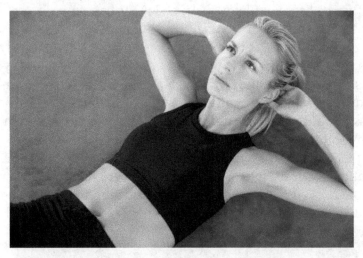

4) <u>Combine meditation with your daily activities</u>. This way you can turn anything you are doing into a mindful meditation. For instance, if you are cleaning the house, notice how you feel as you perform this task; pay attention to the way you move or to the sensation of the objects in your hands. When you are in the car, notice how you feel as you sit in your seat or put your hands on the steering wheel. Once you start driving, pay attention to your feelings and thoughts as you drive through traffic, pay a toll, or hear horns honking around you. Or suppose you step into a sauna or take a warm bath. You can notice how you are caring for your body, as you feel the water or put soap around your body. And if you are lying in bed in the morning before you get up or at night before you fall asleep, you can focus on different parts of your body and notice the sensations, thoughts, and feelings that come up for you. In short, whatever you are doing, you can apply these meditation techniques. Doing so will help to make you calmer as well as more aware of yourself and your surroundings.

Importantly, whenever you focus on being mindful, remain in the present. Should you feel your attention drift, put your focus back on your breathing. As you do, notice what you are thinking or feeling, and do so without any judgment. Don't try to analyze and think about what you should or shouldn't be thinking or feeling. Just accept your thoughts and feelings for whatever they are, and stay grounded and centered in the present.

Some Additional Considerations for Using Mindful Meditation

Here are some additional thoughts in response to common questions that may come up for as you start practicing with these techniques.

- You can engage in these meditation activities at any time, although an ideal time to meditate is in the morning after you wake up. This is a good way to begin your day feeling relaxed and energetic. Also, you can engage in some meditation in the morning, on a break during the day, and at night before you go to sleep, which can make your sleep especially restful.

- There is no right time on how long you should meditate. This meditation time varies for different people, and you should do what feels right for you. When you first meditate, try beginning with 10 minutes at a time, and gradually increase the time you meditate as you get more comfortable with the process. A common time for many people is 20 to 30 minutes, though some people meditate for up to 60 minutes. You can also split up the time you meditate into two or three shorter sessions. It's a good idea to use a timer, as previously mentioned, so you don't have to pay attention to the time, which can break up your session. Another good idea is to take your phone off the hook or turn it off, so you don't get any calls during your session.

- If you have trouble concentrating, a good way to regain your focus is to concentrate on your breathing. Don't worry if any distractions occur. Just remind yourself to focus again and return your attention to your breathing. Or you might concentrate on one or more of your senses, such as any sounds you hear around you, such as the hum of an air conditioner if you are inside or the wind blowing through the trees if you meditate outdoors. And don't be critical of yourself, because you are not being tested or performing for an audience. You are just doing this meditation for yourself.

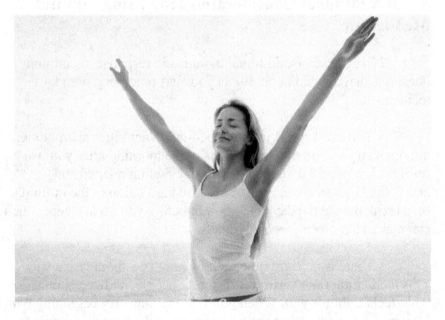

- To help you concentrate in the beginning, limit the number of things you try to be aware at the same time. For example, start with what you see around you, and then add in another sense to pay attention to. To illustrate, suppose you gaze at a flower that's in front of you or in your mind's eye. At first you might pay attention to the colors and shape of the petals and leaves. Then you might add your sense of smell, so you notice how the flower smells. Additionally, you might add the sense of touch, as you feel the petals, leaves, and stems.

- Sometimes you may wonder if you might use meditation to get answers to questions. The answer is that you can use a different type of meditation to do this, such as when you go on a journey to get answers. But in Mindful Meditation, the goal is to just relax and get rid of any stress in your life. Thus, it's better not to try to think about anything. Rather, only focus on your breathing, and if any thoughts come to you, turn your attention away from them and focus back on your breath.

- To help you keep your concentration, focus your attention on something present in the current moment. Ideally, focus on your breath, but you can turn your attention to a background noise or to the sensations of your body. Don't worry if you mind drifts off to think about an experience you had that day, a past memory, or anything else. Just notice that your mind has drifted and refocus on your breathing, background noise, bodily sensations, or something else that you use for your focus. And don't criticize yourself for letting your mind drift. It's common for this to happen, especially when you first start to meditate. Just refocus your attention and let any thoughts go. You'll discover that the more you continue your meditation practice, the easier and easier it will be to regain your focus and let go of any thoughts by observing them without responding to them. In this way, you can let any distrations flow by like they are a passing cloud, stream of water, or leaf blowing in the wind.

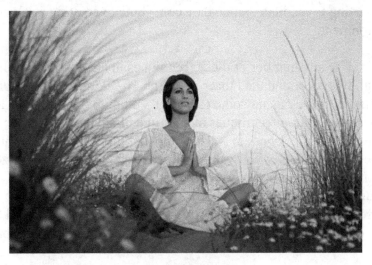

- Once you learn how to concentrate in these sessions, you will find that Mindful Meditation provides you with a series of benefits. These include reducing your feelings of stress, controlling your emotional feelings and how you respond to others, improving your communication with others, and making you more productive. Mindful Meditation provides these benefits, described in more detail in the discussion of why you should meditate, because it helps you stay focused and relax, which contributes to the reduction in stress. Should you feel really depressed about something, meditation may not get rid of this feeling entirely, since you probably need more therapeutic help. But meditation can reduce your feelings of despair, so you are better able to get rid of such depressed feelings with additional help. Moreover, meditation can help you communicate better, because you will be able to be more attentive to those you communicate with, so you will be more conscious and considerate when you speak with them. In fact, the findings of scientists and researchers show that Mindful Meditation, along with other types of meditation, does increase your physical and mental health.

- While many people prefer to meditate in a quiet room, you can also listen to soothing music, sounds from nature, or a very low combination of sounds called "white noise" to help with concentration. These soft sounds can be especially helpful when you are starting to meditate, since they contribute to creating a relaxing environment.

Use any number of these techniques in any combination, though it is recommended that you spend 10-30 minutes three or four times a week using some form of meditation. You can use any of these meditation techniques at any time, though some people like to have a specific schedule, such as meditating for 10 to 20 minutes in the morning soon after waking up to feel focused and energized to begin the day. Others like to scatter their time to meditate throughout the day, whereby they meditate for 5 to 10 minutes before engaging in a particular activity, since they feel that will help them do a better job at whatever they are doing. Still other people like to end their day with a meditation, in which they reflect back and process the events of the day, as they gain inspiration and learning from their reflections. Then, too, some people combine meditating for a short time at different times during the day -- in the morning, before certain activities, and at night. Do whatever works best for you, and select the suggested techniques that appeal to you.

Now think of other techniques that might help you meditate, relax, and visualize other things that make you happy.

_____

_____

_____

_____

_____

_____

_____

_____

_____

_____

CHAPTER 7: CONCLUSION

I hope this book helps you reach your goal of living a healthier active life and losing weight. You can also apply these principles to achieving other goals you set for yourself, both in your personal life and at work.

I have described my experiences in life to show you how I was able to overcome a series of challenges in order to achieve my goals. As described in the introduction, I had a number of hurdles to overcome, including losing my father when I was only five and experiencing poverty as my mother struggled with a variety of jobs to keep a roof over our heads. Additionally, I was sexually abused in my childhood, and I felt a lack of self-confidence and self-worth, which led me to overeat to feel good. But that overeating only contributed to a vicious cycle in which I felt worse about my self-image, which led me to eat more and feel worse about myself, until I weighed 220 pounds.

Then, as I described, I got the motivation to make a change in my life after hearing an Oprah Winfrey program about setting goals to achieve your dreams and after reading a series of self-help books. After that, enrolling at a local YMCA and participating in weight loss and strength building programs made all the difference. I began to eat better and to exercise, and the pounds rolled off. In the process, I kept feeling better about myself, and then I wanted to help others achieve the same kind of success that I did.

As a result, I wrote this book, which shows what I learned about the power of exercise, the importance of eating a good breakfast, and knowing how you burn calories, so you can adjust your eating patterns to take advantage of this knowledge. The basic principle is that the body first burns sugars, then fats, and finally protein. Therefore, you want to eat so that you have the proper balance of sugars and fats available in order to burn as little protein as possible. I also discovered the importance of meditation to help stay centered and grounded.

After discussing what I learned, the book has focused on the major elements of a good weight loss and strength building program to stay healthy and fit. I can't emphasize this principle enough. You should start the day with a good healthy breakfast, since that will give you the energy to accomplish whatever you want that day. It will contribute to your eating less in your other meals. And it will give you the sugars and fats you need, so you burn those first.

Next I discussed how to increase your strength as well as lose weight as you burn calories by lifting weights. You will find a weight lifting program of about 20-30 minutes a day is ideal. You can work your way up from starting with five pound weights, and as you gain muscles and strength, you can lift even more. You will also find doing push-ups is another way to build your strength and your muscles. This kind of exercise is called anaerobic exercise, whereas when you run or walk, this is aerobic exercise, which is good for your heart. It's good to combine both types of exercise, and you can adjust what you eat, so you eat relatively more or less sugars or fats in your diet, because you burn your calories in different ways, depending on what exercises you do and how intensely you do them.

This process of dieting and exercising in a certain way can seem fairly complicated, which is why it's important to understand how your body burns carbs and proteins. A number of scientists and researchers have explored the biology and chemistry of what happens in your body, and knowing this can help you see the reason for eating and exercising in a certain way.

Finally, I have recommended a series of meditation techniques, because I have found meditation extremely helpful in everything you do. It can help you get more relaxed, set goals, focus on accomplishing them, and see yourself becoming healthier and more fit as you continue on this weight loss and strength building program. Meditation can also help you overcome any challenges you face during the day, whether they are related to your health and fitness goals or affect anything else in your life.

My hope is that you will find all of these approaches to eating better, becoming healthier, losing weight, and meditating as helpful as I have found them. And you have my best wishes for reaching your goals.

You'll see a workbook in the Appendix, where you can track your progress by recording your plans for losing weight and building your strength. You can also begin a daily journal of what you do and your progress.

I'm so glad that you have gotten my book, and if you want to read more, I have included a reference guide to other books and articles. I welcome your feedback, and I'm especially interested in learning what else you might like me to write about to help you create a healthier you. Some possibilities might include participating in different types of exercise programs or ways to feel happier and satisfied in life generally. Just write to me and let me know what you are interested in, and if enough of you are interested, that will be the subject of my next book.

APPENDIX

A WORKBOOK TO TRACK YOUR PROGRESS

The following workbook is designed to help you chart your progress.

MY PLANS FOR LOSING WEIGHT AND BEING FIT

Nutrition

1) Foods I plan to eat for my weight loss program.

2) Foods I plan to avoid

Exercises

1) Aerobic exercise (such as running, walking) I plan to engage in

2) Anaerobic exercises (such as push-ups, lifting weights) I plan to engage in

3) Other things I plan to do to be active

Time Devoted to Fitness Activities

1) How much time each day or week I plan to devote to these activities

2) What times do I plan to engage in these fitness activities

3) Where do I plan to engage in these activities (ie: join a gym, exercise at home, take a class,
    participate with friends)

What Do I Plan to Do to Improve Other Areas of My Life

1) Work

2) In relationships with family members

3) In relationships with others

MY DAILY JOURNAL OF LOSING WEIGHT AND BEING FIT

This is where to record your activities at the end of the day, along with your thoughts about how you are doing and what you need to do. Be sure to reward yourself from time and time as you achieve accomplishments along the way. Add in your own dates for each day. Continue adding to the schedule.

Week 1:_____

Day 1_____

Day 2_____

Day 3_____

Day 4_____

Day 5_____

Day 6_____

Day 7_____

Week 2:_____

Day 8_____

Day 9_____

Day 10_____

Day 11_____

Day 12_____

Day 13_____

Day 14_____

CHARTING MY PROGRESS

For each day, note your progress. You can create an Excel file to do this with these headings:

- Date
- Breakfast (est. calories)
- Lunch (est. calories)
- Dinner (est. calories)
- Snacks (est. calories)
- Weight (pick the same time each day, since weight varies over day;
    when you wake up is best)
- Aerobic Exercises
    - Running - Time
    - Dancing - Other
    - Other (specify) - Time
- Anaerobic Exercises
    - Pushups - Time
    - Lifting Weights - Time
    - Other (specify) - Time
- Other Activities (specify) - Time
- Muscle Measurements
    - Arms
    - Legs
- Other changes in my life
    - At work
    - With my family
    - In Other Relationships

REFERENCES AND RESOURCES

This section features the books I have referenced in researching and writing this book. I have divided this section into these categories:

- Books on Dealing with Overeating and Being Overweight,
- Books on Recommended Psychological and Self-Help Techniques for Overcoming the Mental, Emotional, and Spiritual Blocks to Personal Healing.

I have organized the books in each category in reverse chronological order, with the latest book first. I have also added some general observations about these books.

BOOKS

Books about Overeating and Being Overweight

This is an extremely popular category, which includes both personal journeys and self-help books that emphasize the psychology of overcoming the problem of overeating and being overweight. Several use the Mindful Meditation approach. Almost all of the authors are women, who describe their own journey or their work in counseling others, though there are a few male authors who are psychologists and counselors. While most books are independently published or from small presses, a number of books have been published by traditional publishers who specialize in self-help books, such as New World Library, Hay House, New Harbingers, Rodale, Adams Media, and Conari Press. Some of their books have done very well, even those published over five years ago. A few independently published books have sold well, too.

Compulsive Overeating: How to Stop Obesity and Emotional and Binge Eating Disorder by Developing Long-Term Intuitive Healthy Mindfulness Habits by Ashley Brain. Independently Published, 2020. 180 pages. Amazon Rank, Paperback: 713,835; Kindle: 276,472.

Whole Person Integrative Eating: A Breakthrough Dietary Lifestyle to Treat the Root Causes of Overeating, Overweight, and Obesity by Deborah Kesten. White River Press, 2020. 308 pages. Amazon Rank, Paperback: 1,356,976.

Sweet Journey to Transformation: Practical Steps to Lose Weight and Live Healthy by Teresa Shields Parker. Write the Vision, 2019. 258 pages. Amazon Rank: Paperback: 752,940.

It's All About Calories: How to Eat What You Want and Lose Weight Immediately by Gabrielle Hollis. Amazon.Com Services, 2019. 69 pages. Amazon Rank, Kindle: 779,126.

The Binge Cure: 7 Steps to Outsmart Emotional Eating by Nina Savelle-Rocklin. Dr. Nina, Inc.2019. 188 pages. Amazon Rank, Paperback: 258,672.

When Food Is Comfort: Nurture Yourself Mindfully, Rewire Your Brain, and End Emotional Eating by Julie M. Simon. New World Library, 2019. 356 pages. Amazon Rank: Paperback: 25,207.

Facing Overweight and Obesity: A Complete Guide for Children and Adults by Fatima Cody Standford. MGH Psychiatry Academy, 2019. 358 pages. Amazon Rank, Kindle: 363,365.

Diagnosing and Treating Overweight and Obese Patients by John Whyte. NetCe, 2018. 85 pages. Amazon Rank, Kindle: 909,741.

Not Your Average Runner: Why You're Not Too Fat to Run and the Skinny on How to Start Today by Jill Angie. Morgan James Publishing, 2018. 132 pages. Amazon Rank, Paperback: 134,690.

The Overweight Brain by Lois Holzman. CreateSpace, 2018. 204 pages. Amazon Rank, Paperback: 211,566.

Starving in Search of Me: A Coming-of-Age Story of Overcoming an Eating Disorder by Marissa LaRocca. Mango, 2018. 214 pages. Amazon Rank, Paperback: 808,751.

Helping Patients Outsmart Overeating: Psychological Strategies for Doctors and Health Care Providers by Karen R. Koenig and Paige O'Mahoney, MD. Rowman & Littlefield, 2017. 260 pages. Amazon Rank, Hardcover: 1,759,256.

The Food Addiction Recovery Workbook: How to Manage Cravings, Reduce Stress, and Stop Hating Your Body by Carolyn Coker Ross, MD. New Harbinger Publications, 2017. 240 pages. Amazon Rank, Paperback: 181,360.

Brain-Powered Weight Loss: The 11-Step Behavior-Based Plan that Ends Overeating and Leads to Dropping Unwanted Pounds for Good by Eliza Kingsford. Rodale Books, 2017. 256 pages. Amazon Rank, Hardcover: 141,181.

The Overweight Mind: The Undeniable Truth Behind Why You're Not Losing Weight by Jay Nixon. CreateSpace, 2017. 154 pages. Amazon Rank, Paperback: 452,735.

The Emotional Eating Workbook: A Proven-Effective, Step-by-Step Guide to End Your Battle with Food and Satisfy Your Soul by Carolyn Coker Ross. New Harbinger Publications, 2016. 216 pages. Amazon Rank, Paperback: 61,659.

Accidentally Overweight: The 9 Elements that Will Help You Solve Your Weight-Loss Puzzle by Dr. Libby Weaver. Hay House, 2016. 256 pages. Amazon Rank, Paperback: 628,789.

Mini Habits for Weight Loss: Stop Dieting. Form New Habits. Change Your Lifestyle without Suffering by Stephen Guise. Selective Entertainment, 2016. 252 pages. Amazon Rank, Paperback: 25,802.

The Mindfulness-Based Easting Solution: Proven Strategies to End Overeating, Satisfy Your Hunger, and Savor Your Life by Lynn Rossy. New Harbinger Publications, 2016. 232 pages. Amazon Rank, Paperback: 107,585.

Never Binge Again: Reprogram Yourself to Think Like a Permanently Thin Person. Stop Overeating and Binge Eating and Stick to the Food Plan of Your Choice! By Glenn Livingston. CreateSpace, 2015. 162 pages. Amazon Rank, Paperback: 9,353.

Over 50, Overweight & Out of Breath: A Year of Going from Super Fat to Super Fit by Laura E. Sinclair. CreateSpace, 2013. 134 pages. Amazon Rank, Paperback 803,886.

End Emotional Eating: Using Dialectical Behavior Therapy Skills to Cope with Difficult Emotions and Develop a Healthy Relationship to Food by Jennifer Taitz. New Harbinger Publications, 2012. 256 pages. Amazon Rank, Paperback: 257,247.

Stop Eating Your Heart Out: The 21-Day Program to Free Yourself from Emotional Eating by Meryl Hershey Beck. Conari Press, 2012. 256 pages. Amazon Rank, Paperback: 183,092.

Overcoming Overeating: How to Break the Diet/Bing Cycle and Live and Healthier, More Satisfying Life by Jane R. Hirschmann. CreateSpace, 2010. 316 pages. Amazon Rank: Paperback: 829,197; Kindle: 152,457.

The End of Overeating: Taking Control of the Insatiable American Appetite by David A. Kessler. Rodale Books, 2010. 352 pages. Amazon Rank, Paperback: 27,811.

Till the Fat Girl Sings: From an Overweight Nobody to a Broadway Somebody: A Memoir by Sharon Wheatley. Adams Media, 2006. 256 pages. Amazon Rank, Paperback: 663,379.

The Binge Eating and Compulsive Overeating Workbook: An Integrated Approach to Overcoming Disordered Eating by Carolyn Ross. New Harbinger Publications, 2009. 256 pages. Amazon Rank, Paperback: 136,024.

Inside Out: Portrait of an Eating Disorder by Nadia Shivack. Atheneum Books for Young Readers, 2007. 64 pages. Amazon Rank, Hardcover: 1,354,960.

Books about Recovering from Trauma Generally

Only a few books deal with overcoming trauma from a variety of sources, and most of these are from traditional publishers, and some of the recent ones have done very well -- under 20,000 in ranking. The approach is from a self-help or inspirational perspective, emphasizing what to do to heal yourself.

Satisfied: A 90-Day Spiritual Journey Toward Food Freedom by Dr. Rhona Epstein. Dexterity, 2018. 224 pages. Amazon Rank, Paperback: 15,557.

The Body Keeps the Score: Brain, Mind, and Body in the Healing of Trauma by Bessel van der Kolk, MD. Penguin Books, 2015. 464 pages, Amazon Rank, Paperback: 27.

Recovering from Sexual Abuse, Addictions, and Compulsive Behaviors: "Numb" Survivors by Sandra L. Knauer. Routledge, 2014. 398 pages. Amazon Rank, Kindle: 1,864,243.

Recover to Live: Kick Any Habit, Manage Any Addiction: Your Self-Treatment Guide to Alcohol, Drugs, Eating Disorders, Gambling, Hoarding Smoking, Sex and Porn by Christopher Kennedy Lawford. BenBella Books, 2014. 352 pages. Amazon Rank, Paperback: 640,082.

ARTICLES

Articles about Eating a Good Breakfast

Behan, Mollie, "Benefits of Breakfast," University of New Hampshire, Healthy UNH, https://www.unh.edu/healthyunh/blog/2014/05/benefits-breakfast

"Breakfast," Better Health, https://www.betterhealth.vic.gov.au/health/healthyliving/breakfast

"Breakfast: Is It the Most Important Meal?" *WebMD,* December 27, 2018. https://www.webmd.com/food-recipes/breakfast-lose-weight

Brown, Jessica. "Is Breakfast Really the Most Important Meal of the Day?" *BBC.com*, November, 2018. https://www.bbc.com/future/article/20181126-is-breakfast-good-for-your-health

Ducharme, Jamie, "Is Breakfast Really Good for You? Here's What the Science Says," *Time,* January 30, 2019. https://time.com/5516364/is-eating-breakfast-healthy

Newman, Dennis, "The Benefits of Eating Breakfast," *WebMD,* December 27, 2018. https://www.webmd.com/diet/features/many-benefits-breakfast

"7 Reasons Why Breakfast Really Is the Most Important Meal of the Day," *Mental Floss,* https://www.mentalfloss.com/article/80160/7-reasons-why-breakfast-really-most-important-meal-day

"6 Reasons Why Breakfast Is the Most Important Meal of the Day," *UMPC Health Beat,* July 9, 2017. https://share.upmc.com/2017/07/reasons-breakfast-is-important

"The Science Behind Breakfast," Rush: Health and Wellness, https://www.rush.edu/health-wellness/discover-health/why-you-should-eat-breakfast

"Why Is Breakfast Important?" *Shake Up Your Wakeup,* http://www.shakeupyourwakup.com/why-is-breakfast-important

Articles about Strength Training

Barnett, Ann; Smith, Ben; Lord, Stephen R. ; Williams, Mandy; and Baumand, Adrian, "Community-based Group Exercise Improves Balance and Reduces Falls in At-Risk Older People: A Randomised Controlled Trial", *PubMed*, July, 2003. https://pubmed.ncbi.nlm.nih.gov/12851185

Canter, Len, "The Surprising Benefits of Weight Training," MedicalXPress, October 11, 2019. https://medicalxpress.com/news/2019-10-benefits-weight.html

Chai, Carmen, "8 Reasons Why Weight Training Is Incredible for Your Health," *Global News* June 12, 2017. https://globalnews.ca/news/3513498/8-reasons-why-weight-training-is-incredible-for-your-health

Del Turco, "11 Benefits of Strength Training That Will Convince You to Lift Weights," LiveStrong.com, April 22, 2020.

https://www.livestrong.com/slideshow/1008208-13-benefits-weightlifting-one-tells/

Gustafson, Kristin, "5 Benefits of Weight Training," Active.com, https://www.active.com/fitness/articles/5-benefits-of-weight-training

Iliades, Chris, MD, "7 Ways Strength Training Boosts Your Health and Fitness," *Everyday Health,* May 13, 2019. https://www.everydayhealth.com/fitness/add-strength-training-to-your-workout.aspx

Waehner, Paige, "Why You Should Life Weights and Strength Train," *Very Well Fit,* March 11, 2020. https://www.veryhwellfit.com/top-reasons-to-lift-weights-1231112.
Williams, Lucia "7 Unexpected Benefits of Strength Training for Women," Lucia Williams Personal Trainer, https://luciawilliams.com/7-unexpected-benefits-strength-training-women.

Articles about How Your Body Burns Fuel for Energy

Blonz, Ed, "How the Body Burns Fuel During Exercise," Active.com, https://www.active.com/articles/how-the-body-burns-fuel-during-exercise

Braverman, Jody, "Do Carbs or Protein Burn First?" *SF Gate, Healthy Eating,* November 28, 2018. https://healthyeating,.sfgate.com/carbs-protein-burn-first-11980.html

"The Right Way to Burn Fat, Not Muscle," ISSA, https://www.issaonline.com/blog/index.cfm/2017/the-right-way-to-burn-fat-not-muscle

"Understanding Carbs, Proteins, and Fats and How the Body Burns Them," VirtualMedStudent.com. http://www.virtualmedstudent.com/links/healthy_living/understanding_how_the_body_burns_carbs_proteins_fats_simple.html

"WHere Does Body Fat Go When You Lose Weight?" Cleveland Clinic, January 17, 2019. https://health.clevelandclinic.org/where-does-body-fat-go-when-you-lose-weight

AUTHOR INFORMATION

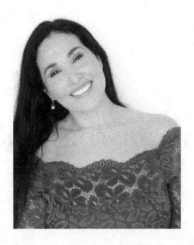

A'Cora Berry was born and raised in Mexico, but moved to the U.S. when she was 17 to find better opportunities. She has acted in several short films, which inspired her to become an assistant producer of several films and write a script for a new film.

A'Cora started her own company MacBe Entertainment at age 37 with the goal of creating films that inspire people and to further other actors' careers. MacBe was named after her daughters, Mackenzie and Bella, her biggest inspirations.

She loves to listen to classical music, read, and act in films. She lives in Rancho Palos Verdes with her husband, their two wonderful daughters, and two mischievous doggies.

CONTACT INFORMATION

A' Cora Berry
Rancho Palos Verdes, California
acoraberry@gmail.com
www.acoraberry.com

ENDNOTES

[1] Jessica Brown, "Is Breakfast Really the Most Important Meal of the Day?" BBC.com, November, 2018. https://www.bbc.com/future/article/20181126-is-breakfast-good-for-your-health

[22] Ibid

[3] Ibid.

[4] Ibid.

[5] "Breakfast," Better Health, https://www.betterhealth.vic.gov.au/health/healthyliving/breakfast.

[6] Ibid.

[7] "The Science Behind Breakfast," Rush: Health and Wellness, https://www.rush.edu/health-wellness/discover-health/why-you-should-eat-breakfast

[8] Mollie Behan, "Benefits of Breakfast," University of New Hamspshire, Healthy UNH, https://www.unh.edu/healthyunh/blog/2014/05/benefits-breakfast

[9] "The Science Behind Breakfast," Rush: Health and Wellness, https://www.rush.edu/health-wellness/discover-health/why-you-should-eat-breakfast

[10] Carmen Chai, "8 Reasons Why Weight Training Is Incredible for Your Health," Global News June 12, 2017. https://globalnews.ca/news/3513498/8-reasons-why-weight-training-is-incredible-for-your-health

[11] Carmen Chai, "8 Reasons Why Weight Training Is Incredible for Your Health," Global News June 12, 2017. https://globalnews.ca/news/3513498/8-reasons-why-weight-training-is-incredible-for-your-health

[12] Chris Iliades, MD, "7 Ways Strength Training Boosts Your Health and Fitness," Everyday Health, May 13, 2019. https://www.everydayhealth.com/fitness/add-strength-training-to-your-workout.aspx

10 Anne Barnett, Ben Smith, Stephen R. Lord, Mandy Williams, Adrian Baumand, "Community-based Group Exercise Improves Balance and Reduces Falls in At-Risk Older People: A Randomised Controlled Trial", PubMed, July, 2003. https://pubmed.ncbi.nlm.nih.gov/12851185

[13] Lauren del Turco, "11 Benefits of Strength Training That Will Convince You to Lift Weights," LiveStrong.com, April 22, 2020. https://www.livestrong.com/slideshow/1008208-13-benefits-weightlifting-one-tells/

[14] Carmen Chai, "8 Reasons Why Weight Training Is Incredible for Your Health," Global News June 12, 2017. https://globalnews.ca/news/3513498/8-reasons-why-weight-training-is-incredible-for-your-health

[15] Ibid.

[16] Lauren del Turco, "11 Benefits of Strength Training That Will Convince You to Lift Weights," LiveStrong.com, April 22, 2020. https://www.livestrong.com/slideshow/1008208-13-benefits-weightlifting-one-tells/

[17] Chris Iliades, MD, "7 Ways Strength Training Boosts Your Health and Fitness," *Everyday Health,* May 13, 2019. https://www.everydayhealth.com/fitness/add-strength-training-to-your-workout.aspx

[18] Carmen Chai, "8 Reasons Why Weight Training Is Incredible for Your Health," *Global News* June 12, 2017. https://globalnews.ca/news/3513498/8-reasons-why-weight-training-is-incredible-for-your-health

[19] Kristin Gustafson, "5 Benefits of Weight Training," Active.com, https://www.active.com/fitness/articles/5-benefits-of-weight-training

[20] Carmen Chai, "8 Reasons Why Weight Training Is Incredible for Your Health," *Global News* June 12, 2017. https://globalnews.ca/news/3513498/8-reasons-why-weight-training-is-incredible-for-your-health

[21] Lauren del Turco, "11 Benefits of Strength Training That Will Convince You to Lift Weights," LiveStrong.com, April 22, 2020. https://www.livestrong.com/slideshow/1008208-13-benefits-weightlifting-one-tells/

[22] Ibid.

[23] Carmen Chai, "8 Reasons Why Weight Training Is Incredible for Your Health," *Global News* June 12, 2017. https://globalnews.ca/news/3513498/8-reasons-why-weight-training-is-incredible-for-your-health

[24] Lauren del Turco, "11 Benefits of Strength Training That Will Convince You to Lift Weights," LiveStrong.com, April 22, 2020. https://www.livestrong.com/slideshow/1008208-13-benefits-weightlifting-one-tells/

[25] Lauren del Turco, "11 Benefits of Strength Training That Will Convince You to Lift Weights," LiveStrong.com, April 22, 2020. https://www.livestrong.com/slideshow/1008208-13-benefits-weightlifting-one-tells/

[26] Paige Waehner, "Why You Should Life Weights and Strength Train," *Very Well Fit,* March 11, 2020. https://www.veryhwellfit.com/top-reasons-to-lift-weights-1231112.

[27] Lucia Williams, "7 Unexpected Benefits of Strength Training for Women," Lucia Williams Personal Trainer, https://luciawilliams.com/7-unexpected-benefits-strength-training-women.

[28] Len Center, "The Surprising Benefits of Weight Training," *Medical XPress,* October 11, 2019. https://medicalxpress.com/news/2019-10-benefits-weight.html.

[29] Ibid.

[30] Ed Blonz, "How the Body Burns Fuel During Exercise," Active.com, https://www.active.com/articles/how-the-body-burns-fuel-during-exercise

[31] VirtualMedStudent.com: "Understanding Carbs, Proteins, and Fats and How the Body Burns Them," http://www.virtualmedstudent.com/links/healthy_living/understanding_how_the_body_burns_carbs_proteins_fats_simple.html

[32] VirtualMedStudent.com: "Understanding Carbs, Proteins, and Fats and How the Body Burns Them," http://www.virtualmedstudent.com/links/healthy_living/understanding_how_the_body_burns_carbs_proteins_fats_simple.html

[33] Ibid.

[34] Blonz.

[35] Jody Braverman, "Do Carbs or Protein Burn First?" *SF Gate, Healthy Eating,* November 28, 2018. https://healthyeating,.sfgate.com/carbs-protein-burn-first-11980.html

[36] Ibid.

[37] Ibid.

[38] Ibid.

[39] "The Right Way to Burn Fat, Not Muscle," ISSA, https://www.issaonline.com/blog/index.cfm/2017/the-right-way-to-burn-fat-not-muscle

[40] Ibid.

[41] "The Right Way to Burn Fat, Not Muscle," ISSA, https://www.issaonline.com/blog/index.cfm/2017/the-right-way-to-burn-fat-not-muscle

[42] "The Right Way to Burn Fat, Not Muscle," ISSA, https://www.issaonline.com/blog/index.cfm/2017/the-right-way-to-burn-fat-not-muscle

[43] Ibid.

[44] "The Right Way to Burn Fat, Not Muscle," ISSA, https://www.issaonline.com/blog/index.cfm/2017/the-right-way-to-burn-fat-not-muscle

[45] Ibid.